DEATH WITH DIGNITY

ETHICAL AND PRACTICAL CONSIDERATIONS FOR CAREGIVERS OF THE TERMINALLY ILL

DEATH WITH DIGNITY

ETHICAL AND PRACTICAL CONSIDERATIONS FOR CAREGIVERS OF THE TERMINALLY ILL

PETER A. CLARK, S.J., PH.D.

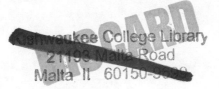
UNIVERSITY OF SCRANTON PRESS

SCRANTON AND LONDON

Library of Congress Cataloging-in-Publication Data

Clark, Peter A., S.J.
 Death with dignity : ethical and practical considerations for caregivers of the terminally ill / Peter Clark.
     p. cm.
 Includes bibliographical references and index.
 ISBN 978-1-58966-214-8 (cloth)
 1. Right to die. 2. Terminally ill. 3. Terminal care--Religious aspects--Christian-
ity. I. Title.

 R726.8.C546 2010
 362.17'5--dc22

                                                                        2010044690

                                        Distribution:

                            University of Scranton Press
                            Chicago Distribution Center
                                   11030 S. Langley
                                   Chicago, IL 60628

TO MY PARENTS, PETER AND MARY CLARK,

MY SISTER, MARY BETH, AND MY BROTHER, PAUL,

WHO TAUGHT ME HOW FAITH, HOPE, AND LOVE

CAN HELP A PERSON DIE WITH TRUE DIGNITY AND RESPECT.

CONTENTS

INTRODUCTION

We are born, we live, and then we die. This is the natural cycle of life. As part of this cycle, death for each of us is inevitable. In fact, as humans we have a 100 percent mortality rate. "Although death is a rite of passage in which we all participate—as family member, provider, or, eventually, patient—we understand little of what is valued at the end of life."[1] In fact, for most of us, we seem to avoid even the mention of death for fear that it might become a reality and we might have to face the inevitable with honesty.

The culture of death has changed over the decades. In the twentieth century, most people died primarily at home and their loved ones, their physician, their minister, priest, or rabbi, and the community assumed responsibility. With the advent of technology and the cultural shift toward individual autonomy, our understanding of dying and death changed. The location of death has shifted to the hospital where the latest advances in medicine and technology are initiated and physicians have become the gatekeepers. Instead of talking about death and dying honestly and allowing individuals to get their lives in order to prepare for the inevitable, today "death is viewed through the lens of biomedical explanation and is primarily defined as a physiologic event."[2] Three false gods have become prominent in contemporary American culture when it comes to any discussion on death and dying: "an unrealistic faith in technology; the view that death is always someone's failure; and a moral sense that pays little attention to clinical realities but veers from wildly lax to painfully scrupulous."[3] These false gods have caused us to avoid the inevitability of death, which has resulted in an unrealistic view of death and the false hope of avoiding it at all cost. The result has been that many individuals are dying without the dignity and respect they deserve. Instead of being surrounded by loved ones with their symptoms adequately assessed and managed, they are often dying alone, alienated, dehumanized, and connected to all types of sophisticated technology that is burdensome and very expensive. The intention of the patient's family and physician is to give the best medical treatment available, but in reality, they are denying the patient the best of care. When the patient dies, it is looked upon, by many, not as part of the natural cycle of life but as a failure of medicine and technology.

When a patient is dying, often there is a silence associated with the dying process. It is this silence that confronts us as we face the fear of the unknown. Instead of going deep within ourselves and confronting the fear and silence, we try to name the silence and even try to circumvent it with the false hope of one last experimental medication or one more surgery or another round of chemotherapy or radiation therapy. Americans have become a "death-denying society," but the truth is that death is a reality that cannot be hidden, ignored, or conquered. It must be faced realistically.

Death is frightening because we are dealing with a fear of the unknown, but it does not have to incapacitate us. If one faces death realistically, surrounded by family and friends, it has the potential of bringing about a metanoia and a transformation for not only the patient but for all who are present. Hopelessness and despair do not have to be the constant companions of the dying patient. Allowing yourself to become dependent on God and others and knowing that you are not alone can nourish the sense of hope. Hope is always present. Preparing for death does not have to preclude hope; it can merely frame it. One can now hope for a lack of pain, a sense of lucidity, good quality of life, and a physician and family who are committed to being there throughout the care process.[4] With this hope, one can now prepare for death, a death that is inevitable, instead of trying to avoid it and hide from it—or even foolishly thinking one can conquer it.

Care for the dying has become a national priority according to many medical associations and the public in general. We now talk about what constitutes a "good death." Is a "good death" one that is à la Jack Kevorkian, or one that happens quickly, or one that the time and place are decided? Or, is a "good death" one that entails hospice care at home or palliative care in the hospital where one's symptoms are relieved, where one is surrounded by loved ones and can prepare for the next stage in life? A "good death" should be one in which the patient and his or her loved ones feel empowered to participate in medical decision making and do what they believe is in the best interest of the patient.

According to studies, a "bad death frequently included scenarios in which treatment preferences were unclear. Patients felt disregarded, family members felt perplexed and concerned about suffering, and providers felt out of control and feared that they were not providing good care. Decisions that had not previously been discussed usually had to be made during a crisis, when emotional reserves were already low."[5] Unfortunately, this is the situation that many terminal patients and their families find themselves in today. Instead of allowing suffering and the dying process to form and inform us, we are allowing it to destroy and emasculate us. "A good death, regardless of the circumstances, means putting medical care in proper perspective and not allowing it to dominate."[6] This notion of a "good death" is not only important to the person who is dying but also for those who survive this event. Therefore, all have a role to play in the dying process: the patient, the family, and the health-care providers.

Dr. Elisabeth Kübler-Ross in the late 1960s formulated five stages that she believed people go through after the diagnosis of a terminal illness: denial, anger, bargaining, depression, and finally acceptance of their inevitable death. She recognized that not all people go through all five stages and, in fact, some could become stuck at one particular stage or move from stage one to stage five, skipping the other three stages. She believed, however, that if one reached the final stage of acceptance, then it was likely that the person would die in peace, which would also give comfort to their family and loved ones.[7]

Understanding these stages and their implications helps not only the terminal patient but family members and even physicians to face death in a realistic fashion. Patients have to be able to talk about their feelings and should be able to allow others to walk with them as they go through the dying process. Family members and loved ones have to be present to the patient in both words and actions, have to respect the patient's feelings and values, and have to be open to learning from this experience. Physicians have the duty to be open and honest with their patients about end-of-life treatment and care, to be willing to hear and respect the patient's feelings and values, and to be there with the patient until the end.

There comes a point in every terminal situation when treatment options become limited or even nonexistent. When a physician can no longer cure, he or she still has the duty to provide care. No patient is ever beyond care. Allowing a patient to die with dignity not only respects that individual patient, but allows us, who are left behind, to learn from this experience so that we are better prepared to accompany others through the same process in the future. Accepting and understanding the dying process will allow patients to die with dignity and respect, will give family members the comfort of knowing that their loved one is at peace, and will give physicians the consolation of knowing that they acted in the best interest of their patient.

To help bring about this notion of a "good death" for all concerned, researchers studying the dying process identified six components of a good death. Even though there is no "right" way to die, these six components can be used as a framework for understanding what patients tend to value at the end of life. The six components are these:

1.   *Pain symptoms and management.* Pain, more than dying itself, is often the cause of acute anxiety among patients and their families.

2.   *Clear decision making.* Patients feel empowered by participating in their treatment decisions.

3.   *Preparation for death.* Patients want to know what to expect as their illness progresses and to plan for what will follow their deaths.

4.   *Completion.* Completion includes not only faith issues but also life review, resolving conflicts, spending time with family and friends, and saying good-bye.

5.   *Contribution to others.* Patients nearing death often achieve clarity as to what is really important in life and are anxious to share that understanding with others.

6.   *Affirmation.* Study participants emphasized the importance of being seen as a unique and whole person and being understood in the context of their lives, values, and preferences.[8]

There may not be a "right" way to die, but what this study does is clearly show that end-of-life care for both patients and families should be holistic, involving not only the physiological but also the spiritual and psychosocial aspects of the process. The problem is that, for this to happen, family members and physicians must be aware of what can be done to help facilitate a "good death."

As a Jesuit priest and—for the past twelve years—the bioethicist for the Mercy Health System in Philadelphia, which includes four acute-care hospitals and one home care service, I have come to see how ill-prepared most patients and family members are regarding end-of-life issues.

In many cases, the patient and family rely totally on their physicians for guidance, but oftentimes the physicians are poorly trained professionally and socially to discuss end-of-life issues and to give advice in the best interest of the patient.

In the course of their medical training, physicians have traditionally been taught how to diagnose disease, to give a reliable prognosis, and to render the appropriate medical treatment. They receive formal instruction in many types of diseases, some of which they will never encounter throughout their medical careers. This becomes even more pronounced when the physician decides to specialize in a particular area. But the one aspect of medical training that all will be confronted with, regardless of their specialty, is the dying patient. Unfortunately, rarely does their medical training prepare them to care for the dying patient and that patient's loved ones.

The curriculum in medical schools and residency programs do an excellent job in preparing these young physicians to heal patients but often fail to incorporate into their training the very practical knowledge they need when the patient is terminal and there is no further medical treatment. This practical knowledge would include areas such as hospice, pain management, palliative care, medical futility, and something as practical as how to give "bad news." As a result of this lack, patients and families are often not given all the viable options regarding end-of-life decisions. Instead, they are encouraged to continue aggressive medical treatments when palliative care would be more appropriate, or they are given a laundry list of options without a complete explanation of what they entail or what the short-term/long-term ramifications are of choosing any one of them.

A more thorough explanation would include issues such as quality of life, quality of function, cost of treatments, long-term disabilities, long-term placement options, and pain. This lack of clarity places patients in a situation where they are often given treatments that are not in their best interest and family members are placed in a situation of watching their loved ones suffer needlessly. Instead of being helpful, decisive, and hopeful to the patient, family members are often helpless, confused, and in a state of despair. At a time when family members are called upon to be present to a loved one in a terminal condition in order to support them and assure them that they will die with dignity and respect, just the opposite happens. Due to their lack of medical knowledge and their feelings of being overwhelmed by the complex world of medicine and technology, family members often feel paralyzed and, in the end, feel guilty that they have abandoned their loved ones at the most crucial time.

Physicians need to be trained not only to be honest with their patients but to feel comfortable with them as they face terminal illness. Those physicians who are comfortable in giving "bad news" view this process as attempting to achieve four essential goals. "The first is gathering information from the patient. This allows the physician to determine the patient's knowledge and expectations and readiness to hear the bad news. The second goal is to provide intelligible information in accordance with the patient's needs and desires. The third goal is to support the patient by employing skills to reduce emotional impact and isolation experienced by the recipient of bad news. The final goal is to develop a strategy in the form of a treatment plan with the input and cooperation of the patient."[9]

To accomplish these goals, a series of six practical steps have been designed to help physicians to deliver "bad news":

1. *Setting up the interview.* Arrange for some privacy, involve significant others, sit down with the patient and family, make a connection with the patient, and manage time constraints and interruptions.

2. *Assessing the patient's perception.* Before discussing the medical findings, the clinician should use open-ended questions to create a reasonably accurate picture of how the patient perceives the medical situation—what it is and whether it is serious or not.

3. *Obtaining the patient's invitation.* While the majority of patients express a desire for full information about their diagnosis, prognosis, and details of their illness, some patients do not. If patients do not want to know details, offer to answer any questions they may have in the future, or offer to talk to a relative or friend.

4. *Giving knowledge and information to the patient.* Warning patients that bad news is coming may lessen the shock that can follow the disclosure of bad news and may make it easier to process that news. When giving medical facts, start at the level of comprehension and vocabulary of the patient. Try to use non-technical terms. Avoid excessive bluntness as it is likely to leave the patient isolated and later angry, with a tendency to blame the messenger of the bad news. Give information in small chunks and check periodically as to the pa-

tient's understanding. Finally, when the prognosis is poor, avoid using phrases such as "There is nothing more we can do for you."

5.   *Addressing the patient's emotions with empathic responses.* When patients receive bad news, their emotional reaction is often an expression of shock, isolation, and grief. In this situation, the physician can offer support and solidarity to the patient by offering an empathic response.

6.   *Strategy and summary.* Patients who have a clear plan for the future are less likely to feel anxious and uncertain. Before discussing the treatment plan, it is important to ask if the patient is ready at that time for such a discussion. Clinicians are often uncomfortable when they must discuss diagnosis and treatment options with a patient whose prognosis is unfavorable. There are various reasons for this, including uncertainty about the patient's expectations, fear of destroying the patient's hope, and fear of their own inadequacy in the face of uncontrollable disease. To overcome these fears, two strategies can be employed: first, exploring the patient's knowledge, expectations, and hopes will allow the physician to understand where the patient is and to start the discussion from that point. Second, understanding the important specific goals that many patients have, such as symptom control and making sure they receive the best possible treatment and continuity of care, will allow the physician to frame hope in terms of what it is possible to accomplish.[10]

Physicians need to have the necessary communication skills to give their patients the information they need in order to make informed decisions, but they also need to have the ability to be a source of support for their patients as they move toward the end of life. Patients want and deserve the truth about their medical conditions, but they want it in a way that fosters confidence, cooperation, and compassion. Basic communication courses in medical school are not enough to address these issues. What is also needed is cultural, social, and spiritual sensitivity on the part of the physician. This is an ongoing process of education that may begin in medical school but needs to be continued throughout residency programs and beyond.

Walking with patients and their loved ones for the past ten years in my dual role has allowed me to witness firsthand the need for some type of practical handbook that will give patients, family members, and health care professionals the information and skills they need in making end-of-life decisions. In addition, walking with my own mother as she died four years ago gave me firsthand knowledge of some of the frustrations family members encounter during the dying process. My sister and I knew the values and desires of our mother in regard to end-of-life medical treatments, and we had the medical knowledge necessary to know what would be in her best interest. Despite this knowledge, we still experienced challenges from the medical staff, a lack of communication and information from her physicians, and conflicting views from various health care professionals that led to confusion.

Luckily, we had the expertise to circumvent many of the pitfalls in the end-of-life care for our mother. But other families, in similar situations, are not as fortunate. Often these families struggle alone with their decisions, and experience confusion and uncertainty as they become lost in the complex world of medicine and technology. At a time when health care professionals should be a source of information and comfort for patients and their families, they are often the cause of their confusion and uncertainty. Instead of feeling comforted and supported at the end of life, these patients and family members often feel abandoned and lost.

This book will attempt to address these complex and often confusing issues in a practical way so that patients, family members, and health care professionals will have some guidance in dealing with end-of-life issues. The focus will be on doing what is medically and ethically appropriate so that patients can die with dignity and respect. To accomplish this task, numerous issues that are pertinent to patients, family members, and health care professionals will be covered in some depth.

Chapter one deals with physiology, consciousness, and the definition of death. Chapter two examines the distinction between extraordinary and ordinary means especially as this relates to feeding-tube issues. Chapter three examines the issue of medical futility and presents a medical futility policy for adult and pediatric acute-care facilities. Chapter four focuses on Do-Not-Resuscitate (DNR) orders, advance directives and living wills, and durable powers of attorney for health care. Chapter five examines pain assessment and management. Chapter six covers palliative care and hospice care. And chapter seven explores the role of spirituality and end-of-life care. The hope is that these topics will give patients, family members, and health care professionals the practical knowledge they need to help terminal patients meet death with dignity and respect.

ONE:
DEFINITION OF DEATH, CONSCIOUSNESS, AND PERSISTENT VEGETATIVE STATE

When does a human life come to an end? Prior to the advent of medical technology, this question was answered rather easily. Death was marked by the permanent and irreversible cessation of the circulatory and respiratory functions. This was known as "clinical death." "This clinical diagnosis was first described in the medical literature in 1959 and was put into practice in the next decade with the use of specific clinical criteria."[1] This traditional concept of death was determined by physicians and was based upon the absence of all vital signs that include cardiopulmonary function—without much consideration given to the role of the brain. In the 1950s and 1960s, new technologies (iron lung, mechanical ventilation, cardiopulmonary resuscitation (CPR), dialysis machines, and the like) made the prolongation of life a realistic possibility. These new technologies posed a unique challenge to the traditional definition of death and in many cases rendered it obsolete.

Death was historically believed to be an event that coincided with the onset of clinical death. With the advent of new technologies, it became understood that death is a process, not a specific event.[2] "In 1959, Mollaret and Goullon used the term *dépassé*, 'a state beyond coma,' to describe a condition from which they believed recovery was not possible."[3] They described the state of irreversible unconsciousness as verified by isoelectric electroencephalogram (EEG) findings. Today, a person can be attached to a ventilator and by traditional standards appear to be alive. The heart is beating, the individual appears to be breathing, and the organs are functioning, but the question remains whether this individual is a living person. "Were these patients simply machine-dependent individuals with a terrible prognosis but still a fragile grip on life, or had they covertly 'crossed the line' that separates life and death, this crossing being simply 'masked' by the technological intervention?"[4]

Whether these ventilated, brain-dead individuals still functioned as living persons—a whole, integrated organism—became a matter of mys-

9

tery and public debate.[5] A prompt reassessment of the definition of death was also stimulated by the need for the harvesting of organs for transplantation. In the 1960s, there was a refinement in surgical transplant techniques and the advancement of cyclosporine and other antirejection medications. Two issues became the impetus for the new "brain death" criteria. "If these patients were already dead, they would be ideal organ donors; and if they were dead, continuing life-sustaining treatment was a grave misuse of our medical prowess."[6] An additional reason for new criteria for determining death focused on the issue of the allocation of scarce medical resources. Maintaining patients on life support for an extended period of time, if they were already dead, was a misuse of those valuable resources. At a time when health care costs began to skyrocket, the issue of allocation of resources, while not explicitly stated, was implicitly understood.

The first formal attempt to address these issues was made by the Ad Hoc Committee of the Harvard Medical School to Examine the Definition of Brain Death. Their goal was to determine the characteristics of irreversible coma and to clarify and standardize medical guidelines for the determination of brain death. They argued that there were two reasons why there was a need for a new definition: "(1) Improvements in resuscitative and supportive measures have led to increased efforts to save those who are desperately injured. Sometimes these efforts have only partial success so that the result is an individual whose heart continues to beat but whose brain is irreversibly damaged. The burden is great on patients who suffer permanent loss of intellect, on their families, on the hospitals, and on those in need of hospital beds already occupied by those comatose patients. (2) Obsolete criteria for the definition of death can lead to controversy in obtaining organs for transplantation."[7]

In 1968, the Harvard Ad Hoc Committee published its report, "A Definition of Irreversible Coma," which proposed a definition and criteria based on whole brain death. These clinical criteria included: (1) unreceptivity and unresponsivity to externally applied stimuli and inner need; (2) absence of spontaneous muscular movements or spontaneous respiration; (3) no elicitable brainstem reflexes; and (4) the presence of isoelectric EEG as a confirmatory value. These conditions had to be confirmed by two separate examinations, twenty-four hours apart.[8] The report argued that patients who passed these tests should be considered brain dead, notwithstanding the continued function of their circulatory system. Since they were dead, all treatment could be stopped and organs—including the heart itself—could be procured even while the heart was still beating.[9]

From 1974 to 1978, approximately half the states enacted legislative statutes or judicial decisions establishing death based on the irreversible cessation of all functions of the brain. The problem was that states were reaching this conclusion through different routes and based on varying legal and medical arguments. There was also a minority opinion still holding the traditional heart–lung-oriented definition, and there were even some arguing for a "higher-brain-oriented" definition.[10] In an effort to reach consensus regarding brain-death criteria, a 1980 Act of Congress established the President's Commission for the Study of Ethical Problems in Medicine and Biomedical and Behavioral Research.

"The President's Commission considered three possible criteria for death: a nonbrain criterion, a whole-brain criterion, and a higher-brain criterion. The first criterion was most consonant with the definition of death as the permanent cessation of the flow of vital bodily fluids, the second with the definition of death as the permanent cessation of the integrated functioning of the organism as a whole, and the third with the definition of death as the permanent loss of what was essential to the nature of man (consciousness)."[11]

The whole-brain criterion was selected. The commission detailed a comprehensive set of clinical circumstances and a battery of tests to identify brain death.[12] "(1) Cessation of brain function is recognized when evaluation discloses findings of (a) and (b): (a) cerebral functions are absent, and (b) brain-stem functions are absent. (2) Irreversibility is recognized when evaluation discloses findings of (a), (b), and (c): (a) the cause of coma is established and is sufficient to account for the loss of brain functions, (b) the possibility of any recovery of the brain function is excluded, (c) cessation of all brain functions persists for an appropriate period of observation and/or trial of therapy."[13]

In 1980, the National Conference of Commissioners on Uniform State Laws formulated the Uniform Determination of Death Act (UDDA) which legally defines death based on the recommendations of the President's Commission. This federal legislation was either enacted or acknowledged in case law by all fifty states. This legal articulation of the whole-brain death criteria states, "An individual who has sustained either (1) irreversible cessation of circulatory and respiratory functions, or (2) irreversible cessation of all functions of the entire brain, including the brain stem, is dead. A determination of death must be made in accordance with accepted medical standards."[14] This has become the legal definition of death in the United States in all fifty states.

The clinical diagnosis of brain death can vary from hospital to hospital, but—after ruling out drug intoxication or hypothermia as causes of a patient's unresponsiveness—the basics are these:

1.   Cessation of cerebral function is attested by deep coma without clinical response to any physical stimuli;

2.   brain stem function is assessed by testing for cranial nerve function, including papillary, corneal, oculocephalic, oculovestibular, and oropharyngeal reflexes;

3.   absence of spontaneous respiration as determined by an apnea test (patient is removed from the ventilator to observe whether spontaneous breathing commences);and

4.   following these clinical tests, laboratory tests will be performed to ascertain total lack of higher brain function. These laboratory tests include EEG, a brain-stem-evoked potentials study, or a cerebral blood flow study.[15]

Confirmatory tests are optional when the clinical criteria are met unambiguously. If specific components of clinical testing cannot be reliably evaluated, these tests are usually repeated between six and twenty-four hours later to ensure irreversibility, with life support being supplied for the interim. The determination of death became a strict technical assessment done by physicians.[16]

Despite the clear clinical criteria for determining brain death, there are cultural and religious groups who do not agree with these criteria. "Various cultural and religious groups (e.g., some First Nation [that is, Native American] and Asian cultures, and Orthodox Judaism) do not accept that death has occurred until all vital functions have ceased."[17] The Orthodox Jews still hold to a heart–lung standard of death on religious grounds. To accommodate such beliefs, the New York State Hospital Review and Planning Council in 1987 adopted regulations developed by the New York State Task Force on Life and Law. The Task Force recommended that "hospitals should develop policies, in consultation with community representatives, that would reasonably accommodate the beliefs of those who reject the brain death standard on religious or moral grounds."[18] In 1991, New Jersey passed legislation known as the "Declaration of Death Act" granting an ex ception or "conscience clause" to brain death on religious grounds. The statute has separate sections recognizing "traditional cardiopulmonary criteria" and "modern neurological criteria," and that prohibits the physician from using the latter when he or she has reason to believe that a declaration on the basis of neurologic criteria would violate the personal religious beliefs of the individual.[19]

Bioethicist Robert Olick argues that such a conscience clause "signals a new direction for the development of public policy governing the declaration of death in pluralistic communities."[20] Even though the brain-death standard is widely accepted in the United States, there are still families who demand continued support despite the determination of death, because of grief, denial, or the fact that their loved one appears to look no different today than they did the day before death was determined. Explanations about neurological brainstem functioning does not make much sense to some people who see a warm body with a beating heart. The issue of brain death has become more complicated because physicians often fail to correct a family's misconceptions concerning the brain-death standard or even give them the impression that it is up to them to decide whether the patient is dead or alive.[21]

The term *brain death* is complex because it has medical, legal, ethical, and even religious considerations. If it is confusing and complex for the medical profession, it is easy to see how it is confusing for laypeople. One of the major areas of confusion centers on how families often use the term *brain death* to include those patients who are minimally conscious, severely brain damaged, or in a persistent vegetative state. Patients who are minimally conscious or in a persistent vegetative state are not brain dead because they do not meet the whole-brain criterion. This has been controversial because consciousness and the ability to relate to others and the wider world has been a defining characteristic of what it means to be a human person.[22]

Consciousness was defined by William James in 1890 as awareness of the self and the environment. Consciousness has two dimensions: wakefulness and awareness. Unconsciousness implies global or total unawareness and is characteristic of both coma and the vegetative state. Patients in a coma are unconscious because they lack both wakefulness and awareness. Patients in a vegetative state are unconscious because, although they are wakeful, they lack awareness.[23] The term *persistent vegetative state* (*PVS*) was coined by Jennett and Plum in 1972 to describe a condition of severe brain damage in which the patient in a coma has progressed to a state of wakefulness without detectable awareness.[24] According to the American Academy of Neurology, approximately 10,000 to 25,000 adults and 6,000 to 10,000 children in the United States are diagnosed as being in a PVS.[25] The leading neurological authorities define a persistent or permanent vegetative state as "a clinical condition of complete unawareness of the self and the environment accompanied by sleep–wake cycles with either complete or partial preservation of hypothalamic and brainstem autonomic functions."[26]

In 1991, the Multi-Society Task Force on PVS, impaneled expert representatives from the American Academy of Neurology, Child Neurology Society, American Association of Neurological Surgeons, American Neurological Association, and the American Academy of Pediatrics to gather and analyze all data on PVS. The clinical criteria they established for the diagnosis of PVS are the following:

1. No evidence of awareness of self or environment and an inaility to interact with others.

2. No evidence of sustained, reproducible, purposeful, or voluntary behavioral responses to visual, auditory, tactile, or noxious stimuli.

3. No evidence of language comprehension or expression.

4. Intermittent wakefulness manifested by the presence of sleep-wake cycles.

5. Sufficiently preserved hypothalamic and brainstem autonomic functions to permit survival with medical and nursing care.

6. Bowel and bladder incontinence.

7. Variably preserved cranial nerve (papillary, oculocephalic, corneal, vestibulo-ocular, gag) and spinal reflexes.[27]

A person can be defined as being in a vegetative state at one month after acute traumatic or nontraumatic brain injury, and present for at least one

month in degenerative/metabolic disorders or developmental manifestations.[28]

The diagnosis of PVS on clinical grounds can be made with a high
degree of medical certainty in most adults and pediatric patients after careful, repeated neurologic examinations. This diagnosis should be made by
physicians who, by reason of training and experience, are competent in
neurologic function, assessment, and diagnosis.[29] One of the criticisms lev-
eled against neurologists is that, since there is no definitive test for PVS, it
is difficult for one to ascertain if someone is in a PVS in contrast to being
in a low awareness state or the locked–in syndrome. Patients, who are in a
low awareness state or minimally conscious, according to the Aspen Criteria, have definite but limited and fluctuating awareness of self and their
environment. They may be able to follow simple commands, give appropriate yes and no responses to questions, make intelligible verbalizations,
or move or feel in response to environmental stimulation: avoiding physical
obstacles in a wheelchair, crying in response to the emotional content of
language, pursuing moving objects with their eyes, or responding to threatening gestures.[30] Locked-in syndrome is a state in which consciousness and
cognition are retained but movement and communication are impossible
because of severe paralysis of the voluntary motor system.[31]

The American Academy of Neurology gives three lines of evidence
based on careful clinical and laboratory studies to support the conclusion
that patients in a PVS are unaware of themselves and their environment.

1.   Motor or eye movements and facial expressions in response
        to various stimuli occur in stereotyped patterns that indicate
        reflexive responses integrated at deep subcortical levels
        rather than learned voluntary acts. The presence of these re-
        sponses is consistent with complete unawareness.

2.   Positron emission tomographic (PET) studies of regional
        cerebral glucose metabolism show levels far lower than those
        inpatients who are aware or in a locked-in state. These lower
        metabolic rates are comparable to those reported during deep
        general anesthesia in normal subjects whom all would agree
        are unaware and insensate.

3.   All available neuropathological examinations of the brains
        of patients with a clinical diagnosis of a persistent vegetative

state show lesions so severe and diffuse that awareness would have been highly improbable, given our biologic understanding of how the anatomy and physiology of the brain contribute to consciousness.[32]

An accurate diagnosis is critical for determining PVS. Neurological authorities agree that errors in diagnosis have occurred because of confusion about terminology used to describe patients in this condition, the inexperience of the examiner, or an insufficient period of observation. However, if neurologists are aware of the potential problems in the clinical diagnosis of PVS and are precise and careful when applying the suggested clinical criteria, and if the patient has been in the vegetative state three months after a nontraumatic brain injury (or twelve months after a traumatic brain injury), the diagnosis of PVS can be made with a high degree of clinical certainty that the chance of the patient regaining consciousness is exceedingly small.[33]

Prognosis for recovery can be classified as recovery of consciousness and recovery of function. "Recovery of consciousness can be verified when a patient shows reliable evidence of awareness of self and the environment, consistent appearance of voluntary behavioral responses to visual and auditory stimuli, and interaction with others. Recovery of function occurs when a patient becomes mobile and is able to communicate and learn, perform adaptive skills and self-care, and participate in recreational and vocational activities."[34]

To determine recovery of function the Glasgow Outcome Scale is used. This scale classifies outcomes into five categories:

1. *Good recovery*. These patients have the capacity to resume normal occupational and social activities, although there may be minor physical or mental deficits or complaints.

2. *Moderate disability*. These patients are independent and can resume almost all activities of daily living. They are, however, disabled, as they no longer can participate in a variety of social and work activities.

3. *Severe disability*. These patients are no longer capable of resuming the majority of previous personal, social, and work activities. These patients have limited communication skills

and abnormal behavioral and emotional responses. They are partially or totally dependent on others for their activities of daily living.

4.   *PVS.* clinical condition of complete unawareness of the self and the environment.

5.   *Death.*[35]

One of the most definitive studies on recovery from PVS was done by the Multi-Society Task Force on PVS in 1994. Recovery of consciousness and function was based on a review of 754 cases published in the English-language literature who were vegetative at one month after an acute insult and for whom one-year outcome was available. Emphasis was put on the difference between recovery of consciousness and of function, because although some patients regain their independence, most who are recorded as having "recovered" after months in the vegetative state remain seriously disabled and totally dependent. The data on outcome was given separately for traumatic and nontraumatic cases, and for adults and children.[36]

"The Task Force concluded from analysis of the 754 cases reviewed that the vegetative state could reasonably be declared permanent three months after nontraumatic damage and twelve months after head injury in both children and adults."[37] However, because of the substantial recovery rate for patients vegetative a month after acute brain damage, some guarded optimism is justified during the first three months.[38] The life span of adults and children in a PVS is substantially reduced. For most PVS patients, life expectancy ranges from two to five years. Survival beyond ten years is unusual. The chance for survival of greater than fifteen years is approximately 1/15,000 to 1/75,000.[39] Since recovery of consciousness from a posttraumatic PVS is unlikely after twelve months in adults and children and recovery after three months from a nontraumatic PVS is exceedingly rare, one can determine with a high degree of medical certainty the diagnosis and prognosis of a patient in a PVS after twelve months.

The issue of pain and suffering in PVS patients has also been raised by some who have concerns about foregoing artificial nutrition and hydration. Neurological studies based on "extensive clinical experience, the results of positron emission tomography (PET) studies, and neuropathologic examinations support the belief that patients in a persistent vegetative state are unaware and insensate and therefore lack the cerebral cortical capacity to be conscious of pain. Almost all such patients have some degree of motor activity and eye movement that would be capable of signaling conscious perception of pain and suffering if such existed."[40] Therefore, since PVS patients feel no pain, this concern of added pain and suffering with the foregoing of artificial nutrition and hydration is a non-issue.

Therapy aimed at reversing PVS has not been successful.[41] There have been some reports of benefits from dopamine agonists or dextroamphetamine, but the benefits have been modest at best, and to date there have been no placebo-controlled or double-blind studies.[42] When families accept the diagnosis of PVS, physicians have the responsibility of working with families to determine the appropriate level of care for the patient. There are four levels of treatment: high-technology "rescue" treatments, such as mechanical ventilation, dialysis, and cardiopulmonary resuscitation; medications and other commonly ordered treatments, including antibiotics and supplemental oxygen; hydration and nutrition; and nursing and home care to maintain personal dignity and hygiene.[43]

A rough approximation of the total cost in the United States for the care of adults and children in a PVS is from $1 billion to $7 billion.[44] However, when surrogate decision makers believe that aggressive treatment is not in the best interest of the patient or the patient has an advance directive that states no aggressive treatment including artificial nutrition and hydration if in a PVS, then surrogates have the right to forego all such treatments medically, legally, and ethically, and physicians have the duty—medically, legally, and ethically—to respect the wishes of the surrogate decision maker.

Brain death is a concept that may appear to have clear clinical criteria, but in reality, the clinical criteria are not universally understood and/or applied correctly by medical professionals. The concept of brain death is even less well understood by the general public.[45] Defining death is complex and it will remain a debatable issue. "Confronted with individuals in this seemingly in-between state, we seem to need a 'concept' of death to guide experience; and we seem to need an expertise about the body—standards, tests, protocols, criteria—to discern whether death has occurred in particular cases."[46]

The whole-brain death standard is the best criteria we have to determine death. To expand these criteria to include severely neurologically damaged individuals or those in a persistent vegetative state would open the slippery slope to possibly allowing the harvesting of organs from living human beings or to a subtle form of active euthanasia. Patients in a minimally conscious state or in a persistent vegetative state are categorically distinct from those patients who meet the brain death standard. One is still alive and the other is clearly dead. This does not mean that those who are minimally conscious or in a PVS have to be aggressively treated. After careful ethical discernment, which would include pertinent medical information and consideration of the patient's values and wishes, a decision to not initiate or to withdraw medical treatment would be medically appropriate and morally justified.

TWO:
ORDINARY VERSUS EXTRAORDINARY MEANS:
THE ISSUE OF TUBE FEEDINGS

For five hundred years, the Catholic Church's position on the ordinary–extraordinary means distinction has been the cornerstone for moral decision making when determining if particular medical treatments or procedures were morally obligatory or nonobligatory for individuals. This distinction was based on the prudential judgment of the patient or surrogate on whether the means used offered a proportionate hope of benefit without imposing excessive burdens to the overall quality of the patient's life. The ordinary–extraordinary means distinction was never meant to serve as an abstract categorization of various treatments. Instead, it set up parameters about treatments and then allowed each individual with a well-formed conscience the freedom to make a prudential judgment about what would be in his or her best interest. This understanding of the ordinary–extraordinary means distinction was the standard used in deciding whether a patient or surrogate could refuse to initiate or withdraw ventilators, feeding tubes, dialysis, pacemakers, and so on.

This standard was challenged in 2004 by John Paul II's allocution, "Care for Patients in a Permanent Vegetative State" presented to The International Congress on Life-Sustaining Treatment and Vegetative State: Scientific Advances and Ethical Dilemmas. This single talk opened a debate about the ordinary–extraordinary means distinction and in particular about artificial nutrition and hydration that could have far-reaching consequences. The central core of John Paul II's position is that "the administration of water and food, even when provided by artificial means, always represents a natural means of preserving life, not a medical act."[1] This means that artificial nutrition and hydration for those in a persistent vegetative state is always morally obligatory because, after the latest papal statement, it is now an ordinary means. Failure to provide artificial nutrition or hydration in these cases causes death by starvation or dehydration and, if done knowingly and willingly, is "proper euthanasia by omission."[2]

21

The dilemma is that this single allocution may revise the five-hundred-year-old ordinary–extraordinary means distinction that has guided medical professionals, ethicists, and patients in making well-reasoned moral decisions. Instead of bringing clarity to this issue, this allocution has caused a profound crisis not only for individuals and medical professionals but for Catholic health care in general. Numerous questions are now being asked: Does the Papal allocution apply only to patients in a PVS or to a broader range of patients? Does this statement imply that Catholics may not refuse—either verbally or in their advance directives—artificial nutrition and hydration if they are in a PVS or have a terminal condition? If a patient or surrogate wishes the withdrawal of artificial nutrition and hydration, would the patient either not be accepted in a Catholic facility or have to be transferred to another facility? If a physician continues to provide artificial nutrition and hydration against the wishes of the patient, could the physician be accused of battery or be sued for malpractice? How might the papal allocution impact palliative care programs and hospice programs in Catholic health care facilities? Might insurance companies refuse to pay for what they may deem to be futile treatment? Would families have to absorb some or most of the costs of prolonged care?

The questions raised show the complexity of this issue and the confusion that has resulted. To address these questions and to give clarity to patients and surrogates, the ordinary–extraordinary means distinction will be examined and analyzed in light of the recent papal allocution. What is important to note is that this one statement must be examined in its context and not in a vacuum.

HISTORICAL BACKGROUND OF THE ORDINARY–EXTRAORDINARY MEANS TRADITION

The ordinary–extraordinary means distinction has its origin in the Roman Catholic Church and many scholars believe that it dates back to the sixteenth-century Dominican moralists. There are, however, some who believe it may go back to the fourth century, when St. Basil the Great wrote in his *Long Rules* (Question 55), "Whatever requires an undue amount of thought or trouble or involves a large expenditure of effort and causes our whole life to revolve, as it were, around the solicitude for the flesh must be avoided by Christians. . . . Therefore, whether we follow the precepts of the medical art or decline to have recourse to them . . . we should hold to our objective of pleasing God and see to it that the soul's benefit is assured, fulfilling thus the Apostle's precept: 'Whether you eat or drink or whatsoever else you do, do all to the glory of God' [1 Corinthians 10:31]."[3]

Others argue that it goes back to Thomas Aquinas (1225–1274), a Dominican Friar and Doctor of the Roman Catholic Church. Thomas's belief in the moral measure of all human activity is whether it leads to God, the final end. Thus, if something was "too difficult" or "too burdensome" what was implied was that it might make loving God too difficult.[4] The general obligation to preserve life and the possible limits to that obligation are also influenced by Thomas's concept of God's dominion over the gift of human life, responsible stewardship, and the positive and negative precepts derived from these.[5] Thomas's influence is clearly present, but it is the three Dominican moralists—Francisco De Vitoria, Domingo Soto, and Domingo Bañez—who articulated the foundation of the ordinary–extraordinary means distinction.

De Vitoria (1486–1546) examined the limits of treatment in regards to nourishment and medicinal drugs. In his seminal work, *Relectiones Theologicae*,[6] he states:

> If a sick man can take food or nourishment with a certain hope of life, he is required to take food as he would be required to give it to one who is sick. However, if the depression of spirits is so severe and there is present grave consternation in the appetitive power so that only with the greatest effort and as though through torture can the sick man take food, this is to be reckoned as an impossibility and therefore, he is excused, at least from mortal sin.[7]

De Vitoria is not condoning suicide here. A healthy person may not starve him-herself simply because life is problematic. If the means are effective and not burdensome, then the person is morally obligated to seek nourishment. But if the person is so sick or depressed that eating may become a grave burden, then the person is not morally obliged to eat and does not commit a serious sin. The essential point here is that De Vitoria recognizes both psychological and physiological illness, and his notion of grave burden includes both. In regards to medicinal drugs, he argues that they are not obligatory per se. The obligation to use them rests on the degree of efficacy. One is not obliged to sacrifice one's whole means of subsistence, nor one's general lifestyle, nor one's homeland in order to acquire a cure or obtain optimum health.[8]

It appears that De Vitoria adopted the sixteenth century's version of the "reasonable person" criteria. "To fulfill one's positive obligation to sustain life, it is sufficient to perform 'that by which regularly a man can live.'"[9] The moral components that appear operative here are not natural as opposed to artificial means, but those means that offer a reasonable hope of benefit in regard to cure and return to health. Excessive burdens in terms of financial costs or inconvenience of lifestyle are measured by "the semi-objective standard of the common person regularly considered," or what we refer to as the "reasonable person standard."[10] If the means used to prolong life are ineffective, if the effect is doubtful, or if it involves a grave burden for the person in question, this means need not be morally obligatory.

Prior to the development of modern anesthesia, surgical procedures, especially amputations, were quite painful. Domingo Soto (1494–1560) reasoned that surgery such as amputation of a limb, because of the excessive pain, ought to be considered categorically optional. He argued that such torture was beyond the limits that the "common man" ought to be obliged to suffer for the sake of one's bodily health. Extreme pain can make a beneficial surgery "morally impossible" to bear.[11] Besides the question of pain, Soto also recognizes the role that emotions of fear and repugnance could play.[12] Soto incorporates the dimension of optional versus obligatory, adding that if a procedure or treatment is too painful or burdensome, it is morally optional.

In 1595, Domingo Bañez (1528–1604) was the first to articulate the terms *ordinary* and *extraordinary* regarding obligatory and nonobligatory means of preserving life. He argued that if preserving life was reasonable, it was obligatory, but he insisted that one is "not bound to extraordinary means but to common food and clothing, to common medicines, to certain common and ordinary pain; not, however, to certain extraordinary and horrible pain, nor to expenses which are extraordinary in proportion to the status of this man."[13] One determined if a treatment or medical procedure was ordinary or extraordinary according to whether it was proportionate to one's condition or state in life. "Thus, if something were very costly or burdensome or if it did not offer substantial benefit to the patient, there was no moral obligation to use it. This standard applied to even lifesaving measures."[14]

The Jesuit moralist Juan Cardinal De Lugo (1583–1660) confirms Bañez's position when he writes, "He is not held to the extraordinary and difficult means . . . the 'bonum' of his life is not of such great moment, however, that its conservation must be effected with extraordinary diligence."[15] De Lugo's position, like that of the Dominican moralists, followed the tradition of the Church, which states that human life is a good but not an absolute good. As a relative good, one's duty to preserve it is a limited duty. While a person has freedom over his or her life, one is never permitted to directly take one's life. The issue becomes to what extent one is obligated to preserve one's life.

The traditional understanding of ordinary–extraordinary means remained basically unchallenged until the mid-1900s with the advent of advances in medicine and technology. How to apply the early distinction of ordinary–extraordinary means to issues like oxygen and feeding tubes—especially with permanently unconscious patients—became hotly debated as early as the 1950s. Jesuit moralist Gerald Kelly was one of the first to examine this issue critically. He defined ordinary means of preserving life as "all medicines, treatments, and operations, which offer a reasonable hope of benefit for the patient and which can be obtained and used without excessive expense, pain, or other inconvenience." Extraordinary means would be "all medicines, treatments, and operations, which cannot be obtained or used without excessive expense, pain, or other inconvenience, or which, if used, would not offer a reasonable hope of benefit."[16]

The distinctive element of Kelly's interpretation is that it is a patient-centered, quality-of-life approach consistent with the sixteenth-century Dominican moralists' view. Kelly concludes that no person is morally obligated to use any means, and this would include natural or artificial means, that does not offer a reasonable hope of ameliorating the patient's condition. To clarify this distinction, Kelly was asked if oxygen and intravenous feeding must be used to extend the life of a patient in a terminal coma. He replied, "I see no reason why even the most delicate professional standard should call for their use. In fact, it seems to me that, apart from very special circumstances, the artificial means not only need not but should not be used, once the coma is reasonably diagnosed as terminal. Their use creates expense and nervous strain without conferring any real benefit."[17]

Many believe that the most authoritative historical study on this topic was done by Daniel Cronin (who later became Archbishop of Hartford) in his 1958 doctoral dissertation, "The Moral Law in Regard to the Ordinary and Extraordinary Means of Preserving Life," written at the Gregorian University in Rome. After a review of over fifty moral theologians from Aquinas to those writing in the early 1950s, Cronin concludes that the Church's teaching is consistent in its view: "Even natural means, such as taking of food and drink, can become optional if taking them requires great effort or if the hope of beneficial results (*spes salutis*) is not present." For a patient whose condition is incurable, he writes, "even ordinary means, according to the general norm, have become extraordinary [morally dispensable] for the patient, [so] the wishes of the patient, expressed or reasonably interpreted, must be obeyed."[18]

The importance of Cronin's position is that no means—even food and water—can ever be classified as absolutely obligatory regardless of the patient's condition. Some moralists disputed this fact, however, and claimed that food and water were absolutely ordinary. They even argued that that was what the tradition taught.

On November 24, 1957, in a talk delivered to the International Congress of Anesthesiologists, Pope Pius XII gave papal approbation to the ordinary–extraordinary means tradition that dates back to De Vitoria:

> Natural reason and Christian morals say that man (and whoever is entrusted with taking care of his fellow man) has the right and the duty in case of serious illness to take the necessary treatment for the preservation of life and health. . . . But normally one is held to use only ordinary means—according to circumstances of persons, places, times and culture—that is to say, means that do not involve grave burden for oneself or another. A stricter obligation would be too burdensome for most men and would render the attainment of the higher, more important good too difficult. Life, health, and all temporal activities are in fact subordinated to spiritual ends. On the other hand, one is not forbidden to take more than the strictly necessary steps to preserve life and health, as long as he does not fail in some more serious duty.[19]

Pius XII thus upheld the traditional ordinary–extraordinary means distinction that "involves patient-centered judgments about the quality of life, which must take into account the usefulness of the treatment, one's understanding about death and dying, and the repugnance one may have toward one's life after subjection to a particular medical treatment."[20]

It is also important to note that Pius XII emphasized the importance of viewing the person holistically. In an address given to the International Union Against Cancer in 1956, Pius XII counseled that "before anything else, the doctor should consider the whole man, in the unity of his person, that is to say, not merely his physical condition but his psychological state as well as his spiritual and moral ideals and his place in history."[21] This statement reinforces the traditional understanding of not treating the physiological aspect of the body separate from the person. Benefits of a treatment can only be determined within the context of a person's life.[22] To preserve life at all cost is to risk idolatry and thus would lead a person away from the higher spiritual good which is eternal life.

A contemporary understanding of the ordinary–extraordinary means distinction was given in the 1980 *Declaration on Euthanasia* by the Sacred Congregation for the Doctrine of the Faith. The Declaration follows the tradition on the ordinary–extraordinary means distinction since the sixteenth century, which is based on the effect of the treatment on the patient or those responsible for the care of the patient. The *Declaration* reminds us of the duty one has to care for one's own life and to seek such care for others. But there are limits to this obligation. One needs to judge the means used by "studying the type of treatment to be used, its degree of complexity or risk, its cost and the possibilities of using it, and comparing these elements with the result that can be expected, taking into account the state of the sick person and his or her physical and moral resources."[23]

The Declaration goes on to give four examples: patients are permitted to use experimental, advanced medical techniques, which may be a service to humanity; patients may interrupt treatments if they fall short of expectations; the refusal of a technique that is in use and carries a risk or is burdensome is not equivalent to suicide; finally, when death is imminent in spite of the means used, it is permitted in conscience to make the decision to refuse forms of treatment that would only secure a precarious and burdensome prolongation of life, so long as the normal care due to the sick person in similar cases is not interrupted.[24] Finally, the Congregation for the Doctrine of the Faith reflects the traditional teaching when it writes, "Life is a gift of God, and on the other hand death is unavoidable; it is necessary, therefore, that we, without in any way hastening the hour of death, should be able to accept it with full responsibility and dignity."[25] The only real change is that the document realizes that the terms *ordinary* and *extraordinary* are imprecise as terms in regards to the rapid advancement of medicine and technology. More precise terms would be *proportionate* and *disproportionate*.[26]

Since the issuance of the *Declaration on Euthanasia*, a subtle debate has been underway within some sectors of the Church about how to consider artificial nutrition and hydration, but in reality, it is about how to revise the ordinary–extraordinary means distinction. There are some who are attempting to revise the tradition by arguing that artificial nutrition and hydration are basic care, and therefore always ordinary and morally obligatory, as long as death is not imminent and they can be assimilated by the body. Those arguing that artificial nutrition and hydration can be categorized as ordinary and obligatory are the following: the Pontifical Council on Health Affairs, "Questions of Ethics Regarding the Fatally Ill and Dying," 1981; the Pontifical Academy of Sciences, "Report of the Pontifical Academy of Sciences on the Artificial Prolongation of Life," 1985; the New Jersey Catholic Conference, "Providing Food and Fluids to Severely Brain Damaged Patients," 1987; the Pennsylvania Catholic Conference, "Nutrition and Hydration: Moral Considerations," 1992; and the United States Catholic Conference of Bishops Committee on Pro-Life Activities, "Nutrition and Hydration: Moral and Pastoral Reflections," 1992. Members of these groups maintain that patients in a PVS must be given nutrition and hydration, because these are basic to human life, aspects of normal care, and far from burdensome. They argue that failure to give these patients this basic care results in a new pathology which is starvation or dehydration which leads to death by omission. Their position is that artificial nutrition and hydration is, under most circumstances, normal care and beneficial, and that failure to supply it to patients is intentional killing.

This is a complete revision of the Catholic tradition dating back to the sixteenth century. Traditional moralists made a clear distinction between allowing someone to die and direct killing or euthanasia. The former was always morally permissible; the later was forbidden. Allowing a patient to die included the refusal of nutrition and hydration if these were considered burdensome and nonbeneficial to the patient. This was a broad interpretation of the understanding of benefits and burdens, not the more restrictive interpretation being proposed by the recent revisionists. This controversy is present even in the U.S. Conference of Catholic Bishops fourth edition of the *Ethical and Religious Directives for Catholic Health Care Services* (ERDs). The ERDs provide authoritative ethical guidance for all those working in Catholic health care facilities. The introduction to Part 6 states the more restrictive standard: "These statements agree that hydration and nutrition are not morally obligatory either when they bring no comfort to a person who is imminently dying or when they cannot be assimilated by the person's body."[27]

According to Hamel and Panicola, "In all the opinions we have from the traditional moralists and in all our studies of the tradition, nowhere do we see the exceptional circumstances under which one may morally forego a means for preserving life reduced to imminent death or futility simply because it will not work." For the traditional moralists these were the easy cases. What they strained over and worked out was a practical moral standard for the gray-area cases, of which we see shades of the latter part of ERD Directive 58: "There should be a presumption in favor of providing nutrition and hydration to all patients, including patients who require medically assisted nutrition and hydration, as long as this is of sufficient benefit to outweigh the burdens involved to the patient."[28] In 2009 the United States Conference of Catholic Bishops emended directive #58 to read: "In principle there is an obligation to provide patients with food and water, including medically assisted nutrition and hydration for those who cannot take food orally. This obligation extends to patients in chronic and presumably irreversible conditions (e.g., the 'persistent vegetative state') who can reasonably be expected to live indefinitely if given such care. Medically assisted nutrition and hydration become morally optional when they cannot reasonably be expected to prolong life or when they would be 'excessively burdensome for the patient or [would] cause significant physical discomfort, for example resulting from complications in the use of the means employed. For instance, as a patient draws close to inevitable death from an underlying progressive and fatal condition, certain measures to provide nutrition and hydration may become excessively burdensome and therefore not obligatory in light of their very limited ability to prolong life or provide comfort."[29] The former and present directive follows the traditional understanding of the ordinary–extraordinary means distinction, in which the benefits and burdens are understood broadly relative to the patient. The problem is that this conflict between the broad and narrow interpretation of the benefit–burden calculus was left unresolved, but since the Directive is viewed as having more importance than the introduction, most believed that the broad interpretation was maintained.

It is within this mix that Pope John Paul II's 2004 allocution regarding tube feedings for PVS patients has raised medical, ethical, legal, and even financial implications for all Catholics—and especially for those in Catholic health care today.

IMPLICATIONS OF POPE JOHN PAUL II'S ALLOCUTION

The reason the Pope's latest allocution has caused such a debate and for some people a real sense of moral confusion, is that there appears to be a distinct shift in methodology regarding the traditional understanding of the ordinary–extraordinary means distinction. In the allocution, "Care for Patients in a Permanent Vegetative State," the Pope states,

> I should like particularly to underline how the administration of water and food, even when provided by artificial means, always represents a natural means of preserving life, not a medical act. Its use, furthermore, should be considered *in principle* ordinary and proportionate, and as such morally obligatory *insofar as* and until it is seen to have attained its proper finality, which in the present case consists in providing nourishment to the patient and alleviation of his suffering [emphasis added]. Death by starvation or dehydration is in fact the only possible outcome as a result of their withdrawal. In this sense it ends up becoming, if done knowingly and willingly, true and proper euthanasia by omission.[30]

The medical condition of the patient appears not to be relevant because the Pope declares artificial nutrition and hydration ordinary care that is beneficial. These statements show a complete shift in methodology from the traditional teleological balancing of the benefits and burdens of the impact of the treatment on the patient to a deontological principle that declares artificial nutrition and hydration for PVS patients as ordinary and proportionate and therefore morally obligatory. There is little attention given to person or circumstances.[31] This shift in methodology would appear to reverse the traditional understanding of the ordinary–extraordinary means distinction, dating back to the sixteenth century, which always considered how the treatment affected the life of the patient, the family, and others.

The recent statement of the Pope appears to impact the traditional understanding of the ordinary–extraordinary means distinction in three specific ways. First, the Pope declares artificial nutrition and hydration for PVS patients as "not a medical act" but "normal care." No one is disputing that all people who are ill, whether in a PVS or a terminal condition must be cared for in ways that respect their inherent dignity. "Traditionally, however, this has not meant that food and fluids must always be provided. The traditional moralists understood that even the most common or natural means of preserving life could be extraordinary and hence morally optional."[32] Feeding tubes are used when patients have difficulty in swallowing, have diminished consciousness, or need to supplement inadequate oral intake, when, for a variety of reasons, the patient cannot eat or drink to maintain health or sustain life.

There are several types of feeding tubes. Nasogastric feeding tubes are thin tubes inserted into the nostril, threaded into the nasopharynx, and then advanced down the esophagus into the stomach or into the first portion of the duodenum. Gastrostomy tubes are inserted directly into the stomach, either surgically, or more commonly, by placing an endoscope through the skin. Jejunostomy tube placement can be performed either surgically or with an endoscope that allows the tube to be advanced into the jejunum.[33] Each of these procedures, which carry certain risks of harm attendant to their use, is intended to achieve physiological objectives and requires skilled medical monitoring to assess the effects which clearly constitute a medical procedure. To hold that this is not a medical act or treatment is illogical. In addition, according to Hamel and Panicola, "it seems logically inconsistent to classify nutrition and hydration as basic care that is always obligatory even if artificially supplied, while not doing the same for oxygen supplied by mechanical ventilation or other basic elements of care necessary for life."[34] Consistency in what is regarded as "basic care" seems to be the cornerstone of the revisionists' position. Classifying artificial nutrition and hydration as basic care and not oxygen, which is even more basic to our survival, is not only illogical but is irrational. The Pope's allocution does not give a firm justification for this classification.

Second, the Pope declares that the cessation or interruption of artificial nutrition and hydration leads to death by starvation or dehydration and, if done knowingly and willingly, is euthanasia by omission. The Pope is declaring that the intention of the surrogate, by foregoing artificial nutrition and hydration, is the direct killing of the patient. When a patient needs artificial nutrition and hydration, it is usually as a result of a serious head injury, coma, PVS, or some other neurologic condition, such as a stroke or brain tumor, that prevents swallowing. Death comes not from the lack of tube feeding but from the underlying pathology that placed the person in the condition. The issue here is that the foregoing of artificial nutrition and hydration from a PVS patient does not cause a second pathology —starvation/dehydration, but allows the original pathology to take its natural course of events. The Pope himself, in *Evangelium Vitae*, states, "Euthanasia's terms of reference, therefore, are to be found in the intention of the will and in the methods used."[35] The intention here is not to end the life of the patient but to forego a burdensome treatment and allow the patient to die from the original pathology.

The Pope himself states clearly that euthanasia must be distinguished from the decision to forego what he refers to as "aggressive medical treatment." "Medical procedures which no longer correspond to the real situation of the patient, either because they are by now disproportionate to any expected results or because they impose an excessive burden on the patient and his family."[36] For the surrogate of a PVS patient, the intention is "to recognize that either the proposed intervention is not useful in helping to restore the patient to health or that the patient is dying or in a condition that will lead to death and that the moral obligation is to accompany this person on his or her final journey. The intention might also be to respect the patient's considered wishes when competent not to have such interventions put in place when the patient falls into a persistent vegetative state."[37]

If the intention is to forego a nonbeneficial treatment that the surrogate and the medical professionals believe is disproportionate and not in the patient's best interest, then the intention is to allow the patient to die rather than to terminate the patient directly. These patients will not be abandoned. Instead they will be cared for lovingly, kept warm and clean and treated with the utmost dignity and respect. It should also be noted that, according to the American Academy of Neurology, patients in a PVS do not feel pain, therefore, the withdrawal of nutrition and hydration does not mean a painful death.

Third, the Pope introduces a more restrictive view of the duty to preserve life. The traditional interpretation was a more holistic standard based on the benefits and burdens being understood broadly relative to the person. That tradition held that decisions regarding any means of preserving life must be subject to a benefit–burden analysis. The Pope appears to have reinforced a more restrictive standard based on recent revisions of the traditional teaching by groups like the U.S. Bishop's Pro-Life Committee, in which the benefits and burdens are understood narrowly, apart from relative factors, and nutrition and hydration are given special moral classification.[38] The benefit of a medical procedure or treatment was traditionally viewed as a prudential judgment of the patient or surrogate concerning how a particular treatment or procedure would affect the life of the patient. Benefits and burdens were never judged abstractly. "Not only the means (proposed intervention) but the ends toward which the intervention is aimed are important in moral analysis."[39]

The fact that a particular means was able to sustain a human life did not make such a means beneficial to the person. Traditional moralists did not restrict benefits merely to sustaining life, but included broader, more holistic considerations. Improvements in one's condition, relief of pain and suffering, maximization of comfort, and restoration of health—among others—were all considered beneficial. For DeVitoria and other traditional moralists, the mere preservation of life and vital physiological functions was not sufficient in itself to oblige someone to use a certain means, including food and fluids.[40]

It should also be noted that there is extensive medical literature on the potential harms of tube feedings. There are side effects like terminal pulmonary edema, nausea, diarrhea, abdominal swelling, and impaired consciousness. There are other side effects such as pneumonia and infections at the site of the insertion, and patients often have to be physically restrained from pulling out the tubes.[41] Another burden that had to be considered, according to the tradition, was the expense of the procedure or treatment. The *Declaration on Euthanasia* states that a treatment may be judged to be too burdensome if it imposes an excessive expense on the family or the community.[42] The American Medical Association estimates that the cost of aggressively treating patients in a PVS is anywhere from one to seven billion dollars a year. In a country where approximately 47 million people are uninsured and millions more are underinsured, this seems like a disproportionate expense for the individual, family, and society, when the medical authorities believe there is almost no possibility of recovery after a year.

The traditional understanding of ordinary–extraordinary means was based on treating the whole person, not one part of the person. Just because a treatment could prolong a life did not mean that a particular treatment was a benefit. Benefits must be considered worthwhile both in quality and duration. In the Catholic moral tradition, a medical treatment was beneficial if it restored a patient to a relative state of health. "No matter how long medically assisted nutrition and hydration prolongs the lives of patients in a PVS, it will never improve their overall condition to the point where they can again pursue the spiritual goods of life.[43] Failure to receive a meaningful benefit from a treatment makes that treatment not morally obligatory.

An initial reading of the Pope's recent allocution on tube feedings for PVS patients appears to have introduced a shift in methodology concerning the Church's tradition on the ordinary–extraordinary means distinction. If artificial nutrition and hydration are now ordinary means and morally obligatory for PVS patients, then the implementation of this revision will have wide-ranging implications not only for Catholics but for Catholic health care facilities and their staffs. The purpose behind this statement was to counter the "culture of death" and the attitude of relativism that seems to pervade Western culture. This culture is based on a utilitarian calculus "that would construe human worth on criteria associated with what one can do or achieve rather than who one is."[44] However, while the intention of the Pope's allocution is good, the means to bring about this good may have serious implications that, in the long run, could cause the "culture of death" to be advanced rather than reversed.

THE ROLE OF CONSCIENCE IN MORAL DECISION MAKING

The Pope's statement does seem to narrow the traditional understanding of the ordinary–extraordinary means distinction as applied to artificial nutrition and hydration for PVS patients. Upon a more careful analysis, however, one might interpret this speech as "more of a theoretical clarification, the application of which will have limited clinical or pastoral significance."[45] The reason for this is twofold: first, there are different levels of authority of Church teachings—infallible statements, conciliar documents, encyclicals, congregation documents, apostolic exhortations, allocutions, and so on. The type of document determines the weight of authority the statement holds. For example, a conciliar document such as the *Pastoral Constitution on the Church in the Modern World* or an encyclical such as E*vangelium Vitae* would carry more authority than an allocution.

Thomas A. Shannon and James J. Walter, in an article on this subject in the *National Catholic Reporter*, write,

> Traditionally, allocutions are given to a variety of groups that meet in Rome, but they have not always been seen as the locus for announcing a major political shift. Instead, they have been used by Popes for discussing particular issues, as Pius XII was wont to do. He used allocutions to discuss organ transplantation and the use of analgesics to relieve pain at the end of life. Many of these allocutions were understood to be made in relation to the state of the question in moral theology, and it was well understood that the statements were subject to interpretation by moral theologians.[46]

Thus, the present allocution appears not to be a teaching of a general moral principle but a practical application of the Pope's statement in *Evangelium Vitae*: "In such situations, when death is clearly imminent and inevitable, he can in conscience refuse forms of treatment that would only secure a precarious and burdensome prolongation of life."[47]Teachings of general moral principles carry more weight than a proposal for its practical application. "While the application of general principles calls for serious consideration by Catholics, these do not bind in conscience."[48]

In addition, if one reads the allocution carefully, the Pope does not completely depart from the traditional understanding of ordinary–extraordinary means by making artificial feeding and hydration an absolute requirement with no exceptions. Hamel and Panicola argue that "if the Pope's statement is read in light of the tradition, what he might be saying is that *in principle* nutrition and hydration are ordinary means of preserving life and hence morally obligatory for all patients. . . . Were the Pope going beyond this presumption and arguing instead for an absolute requirement, he would not likely have uttered the phrase 'insofar as and until it is seen to have attained its proper finality.' Here the Pope may be indicating that nutrition and hydration are not always obligatory, but only to the extent that they serve their ultimate purpose."[49] This interpretation would be in keeping with the Church's tradition that human life is a relative good and the duty to preserve it is a limited one. It also is in keeping with the Judeo-Christian tradition that has always walked a balanced path between medical vitalism and medical pessimism.

It seems clear that the Pope was talking exclusively about PVS patients which were the focus of the International Congress at which the Pope read this allocution. As a result, Hamel and Panicola argue, "We may be left with a presumption in favor of providing nutrition and hydration to all patients. But nutrition and hydration can be withheld or withdrawn when they do not attain their proper finality, which for patients in general can be decided on traditional grounds (i.e., holistic benefit–burden calculus) and for patients in a PVS on the more limited grounds set by the Pope (i.e., nourishment and the alleviation of suffering)."[50] This may be true, but because this is an application of a general principle, one could in good conscience, apply the traditional benefit–burden calculus to determine whether to withhold or withdraw artificial nutrition and hydration even for PVS patients. This is accepting the limits of human life, "that a person has come to the end of his or her pilgrimage and should not be impeded from taking the final step."[51]

Second, as with all Church teachings that are not infallible statements, one has the right, with a well-formed conscience, to do what one believes is morally right. The Catholic ethical tradition has always viewed conscience as the ultimate subjective norm of human action. Theologian

Avery Dulles refers to conscience not as a "blind feeling or instinct but a personal and considered judgment about what one ought, or ought not, to do or to have done."[52] To have a well-formed conscience, one has the obligation to search for the truth in a situation by consulting the sources of moral wisdom (scripture, tradition, Church teaching, reason, and experience) and seeking guidance and instruction from those who have knowledge about the particular issue.

It is clear from the best neurological authorities that recovery of consciousness for posttraumatic PVS is unlikely after twelve months for adults and children and recovery from nontraumatic PVS after three months is exceedingly rare for both adults and children. In the event that this diagnosis is confirmed medically, and the surrogate or the patient's advance directive states clearly that the patient would not want extraordinary, disproportionate means used, which includes artificial nutrition and hydration, then examining this situation in light of a broad interpretation of the benefit–burden calculus, said treatment could be withheld or withdrawn as a matter of conscience.

Traditional moralists made a clear distinction between allowing to die—which entails foregoing disproportionate means where death is foreseen but not directly intended—and direct killing by euthanasia. Allowing a patient to die by foregoing aggressive, nonbeneficial treatments is not only morally permissible, but it is treating the patient with dignity and respect. "The decision is based on the fact that physiological existence no longer offers these patients any hope at all of pursuing those goods for which human life is the fundamental condition."[53]

CONCLUSION

The recent papal allocution has caused a serious debate both within the Church and in society as a whole regarding the ordinary–extraordinary means distinction and how it relates to the use of artificial nutrition and hydration. This debate has been instructive not only because death and dying are being openly discussed in a society that avoids such discussions but also because the Pope's concern about moral relativism and a "culture of death" are being examined and critiqued. People are struggling with end-of-life decisions daily and they are in desperate need of guidance. Unfortunately, the media has presented this issue as a papal mandate that is being imposed on all Catholics and, as a result, this has caused much confusion, pain, and even guilt. Some have questioned past decisions to forego artificial nutrition and hydrations and have even wondered if they have committed a sin. End-of-life decisions are difficult enough for individuals and families without adding to their pain and suffering.

Catholic health care facilities are struggling with numerous medical and financial dilemmas without adding another of this magnitude. If taken literally, Catholic hospitals could be in conflict with the law, because they might not always be able to abide by a patient's legal advance directive; they could be in conflict with families, because they might not be able to offer the care the family is requesting; and they could even be in conflict with their staffs, by placing them in compromising positions as a matter of conscience. Fortunately, calmer voices, like the Catholic Health Association, are speaking up and calling for further study and dialogue regarding this issue.

At the present time, our concern ought to focus on the moral relativism in society and the current trend toward a "culture of death." This can be done by respecting the traditional understanding of the ordinary–extraordinary means distinction that has served the Church and society well for centuries. It can also be done by improving end-of-life care by advocating for better pain management, more palliative care centers, and earlier referrals to hospice. The fear is that—if the traditional understanding of ordinary–extraordinary means is abandoned—instead of advocating for a "culture of life," we may end up driving more people toward a "culture of death"—euthanasia and physician-assisted suicide. This would be not only medically irresponsible but morally objectionable as well.

THREE:
MEDICAL FUTILITY

In the previous chapter, the right of a patient/surrogate to refuse medical treatment was examined under the principle of the ordinary–extraordinary means distinction. This constitutional right to refuse medical treatment, which was upheld by the Supreme Court case of *Cruzan vs. Director, Missouri Department of Health* and was extended to the surrogate's interpretation of the patient's wishes, settled one controversy but started another about whether a patient also has a corresponding right to demand medical treatment.[1]

For the past decade, there has been a debate raging within the medical, ethical, and legal communities that has focused on the issue of medical futility. Despite the emergence of medical futility as a dominant topic of discussion, especially as it applies to end-of-life care, the concept is not new. Physicians at the time of Hippocrates recognized some medical conditions as futile and recommended no further treatment for the patient.[2] What fueled the fires of this multifaceted debate has been the patients' rights movement with their perception that the right of self-determination extends not only to the refusal of medical treatments but to demands for overtreatment.[3]

The patient rights movement began as a reaction to the paternalism of physicians who unilaterally overtreated patients and prolonged their lives against their wishes or the wishes of surrogates and family members. The perception of this physician-driven overtreatment resulted in a series of legal cases (ranging from the Quinlan case in 1976 to the Cruzan case in 1990), which gave patients or their appropriate surrogates the legal right to refuse medical treatment, even if this resulted in the patient's death. Despite physician or hospital administration arguments that treatment was appropriate, the courts ruled in favor of the patient's right to determine his or her own medical treatment generally on the condition that there is clear and convincing evidence that the patient would refuse life-sustaining treatment if he or she were conscious and able to do so.

In the 1990s, patients and patient surrogates began to demand treatments that physicians believed were not in the best interest of the patient because they were medically futile and represented an irresponsible stewardship of health care resources. In legal cases ranging from Wanglie in 1991 to Baby K in 1994, the courts ruled in favor of the right of patients or their surrogates to request even those medical treatments from which physicians believed their patients would receive no medical benefit.[4] What has been problematic for the judges in these cases has been the lack of professional or institutional policies on medical futility against which they could judge physician and hospital compliance or noncompliance.[5] These complex cases have set the stage for the present debate over medical futility, which pits patient autonomy against physician beneficence and the allocation of social resources.

Ethically, patients and their surrogates argue that if they have the right to withhold or withdraw certain medical treatments, this also gives them the right to request certain medical treatments because *they* know what is in their best interest. Physicians argue that many of these interventions are burdensome for the patient and medically inappropriate because they fail to achieve the proper physiological effect and result in a misallocation of medical resources. Allowing these treatments compromises the physician's professional integrity, but many physicians feel compelled to comply with the patient's or surrogate's wishes, because they believe that society has mandated the provision of such interventions until patients or surrogates agree to their being withheld.[6]

The ever-present fear of litigation has not only fueled this debate but has placed the very foundation of the physician–patient relationship in jeopardy. This extreme autonomy position ignores the fact that a well-established "best interest" standard assumes both a connectedness of the patient to family and physician and a communication process that allows surrogates to decide based on objective, community-based best-interest standards.[7] To address these concerns, a balance will have to be found that avoids both the traditional physician-driven overtreatment and recent patient or surrogate-driven overtreatment and seeks to balance patient and surrogate rights with physician rights and social justice.[8]

From a legal and ethical perspective, one way to foster this balance would be a process-based approach to futility determinations on a case-by-case basis. The goal of this process-based approach would be a medical futility policy that protects the patient's right to self-determination, the physician's professional integrity, and society's concern for the just allocation of medical resources, and is securely rooted in the moral tradition of promoting and defending human dignity.

LEGAL IMPLICATIONS

Perhaps the greatest challenge in implementing a futility policy is recognition by physicians and health care institutions that adopting a futility policy carries with it the threat of litigation. The state of Texas took the lead in addressing the issue of medical futility from both a medical and a legal perspective. "In 1999, Texas legislation combined three preexisting laws regulating end-of-life treatment into a single law, the 'Texas Advance Directives Act.' This law established a legally sanctioned extrajudicial process for resolving disputes about end-of-life decisions. This mechanism for dispute resolution may be used in response to a surrogate, living will, or medical power of attorney request to either 'do everything' or 'stop all treatment' if the physician feels ethically unable to agree to either request."[9] The Texas law became a model for other states and for individual hospitals seeking to make changes in statutory regulations and institutional policies regarding end-of-life treatment decisions. Futility policies are a relatively new initiative in health care, and there was uncertainty as to how the courts will respond once confronted with a "futile treatment" case.

This changed in March 2005 when Sun Hudson, born with thanatophoric dysplasia, a typically fatal form of congenital dwarfism, was removed from a breathing tube against the wishes of his mother Wanda Hudson. The breathing tube was removed pursuant to Chapter 166 of the Texas Health and Safety Code, the Advance Directive Act. Under this act, the doctor's recommendation to withdraw support was confirmed by the Texas Children's Hospital ethics committee. Although it is not required under the "Texas Advance Directive Act," Texas Children's Hospital took the extra step of getting a judge to rule on their decision. The judge found that the act authorized the hospital to withdraw life support over the objection of the baby's mother.

Wanda Hudson was given ten days from receipt of written notice to find a new facility to accommodate Sun if she disagreed with the hospital decision, but she was unable to find another facility. Texas Children's Hospital stated that it attempted to contact forty facilities, but it, too, was unable to find one willing to accept Sun. On March 15, 2005, physicians at Texas Children's Hospital sedated Sun for palliation purposes, removed the breathing tube and he died within a minute.[10] This was the first time a hospital in the United States allowed the removal of life-sustaining support against the wishes of the legal guardian. It became a legal precedent-setting case that should help relieve the anxiety of physicians and hospital administrators about invoking a medical futility policy in future cases. It appears that the courts acted in the best interest of the patient—who, doctors said, was certain to die and was most likely to suffer before doing so—using a process-based approach.

One of the goals in implementing a futility policy is to facilitate communication between the patient or surrogate and the health care staff so that all parties can come to an acceptable agreement regarding the proposed treatment. If agreement is not reached between the physician or hospital and the patient or surrogate, either party may seek injunctive relief from the courts, or the patient or surrogate may file a medical malpractice action.

Physicians are particularly averse to litigation. The physician who loses a malpractice claim risks damage to his or her professional reputation and the possibility of an increase in malpractice payment premiums. Perhaps even more dreaded though, is the report that will be filed with the National Practitioner Data Bank confirming that the physician lost a medical malpractice suit.[11] A Data Bank report will follow the physician for the remainder of his or her career since all hospitals are mandated to query the Data Bank on a regular basis. Even the physician who prevails in a professional malpractice action expends substantial time meeting with attorneys, answering interrogatories, appearing for deposition and testifying at trial. Obviously then, the threat of litigation alone will deter some physicians from ever invoking a futility policy.

For those physicians who are willing to risk litigation for the sake of preserving their professional integrity, a futility policy does offer legal benefits. Although a futility policy will not insulate a physician from litigation, it should enable him or her to fashion a strong defense in a medical malpractice claim. As a general rule, to prevail in a professional malpractice action, the plaintiff must establish that harm he or she suffered resulted from the physician's having breached the standard of care. A futility policy requires consensus from other physicians and other interdisciplinary committees within the institution that the proposed treatment is not beneficial to the patient. Such a consensus among physicians can then be submitted as evidence in any legal proceedings to demonstrate that the standard of care was not breached.

Implementation of a futility policy may also give rise to claims for injunctive relief. The patient or surrogate may file an action asking a court to order that the "futile" treatment be administered. Likewise, a physician or institution may petition the court for an order that futile treatment not be initiated—or, if already initiated, that it be discontinued, as in the Wanglie case.[12] If the physician has withheld or discontinued treatment in accordance with the institution's futility policy, the court may be more inclined to conclude that the treatment is, indeed, inappropriate.

In the 1995 case of *Gilgunn vs. Massachusetts General Hospital*, the court found that cardiopulmonary resuscitation need not be provided to a patient dying with multiple organ-system failure, even if requested by the patient's family.[13] This case encouraged physicians to examine the issue of medical futility more closely, but the fear of litigation and not being supported by the hospital administration was still paramount.

The need to consider a medical futility policy became apparent when one of the hospitals within our system became involved in a case in which injunctive relief was sought by a surrogate for treatment that appeared to be futile. At the time the treatment was sought, this hospital, which is Catholic, did not have a futility policy. Nevertheless, the case was instructive for us not only because it highlighted the issue of futile treatment, but also because it gave us an opportunity to assess where we stood as an institution when futile treatment is demanded. The type of relief sought in the courts by the patient's surrogate was the same type of relief we can expect patients or surrogates to seek in the future when an agreement on what constitutes futile treatment cannot be reached.

To understand the issue of medical futility, it might be helpful to look at the facts of a particular case. The case in question that convinced us of the need for a futility policy concerned J.L., an 87-year-old semicomatose patient who was admitted several times from a local nursing home to one of our acute-care facilities over the course of a few months. She had been ventilator-dependent, semicomatose, and in multiple-system failure months before she was first admitted to our facility.

J.L. did not have an advance directive and, therefore, her wishes regarding her medical care were unknown to her physicians.[14] She appointed both of her daughters as her health care agents. Regrettably, the daughters had diametrically opposed viewpoints regarding their mother's medical treatment. One daughter, S.A., claimed that her mother wanted to die peacefully and never would have wanted to be dependent on a ventilator. The other daughter, E.L., contended that her mother valued life and would have wanted all available life-sustaining measures employed.

Each time J.L. was hospitalized in our facility, the patient's daughters gave conflicting instructions regarding their mother's medical treatment, leaving J.L.'s physicians in an unmanageable legal (and ethical) position. In one instance, when J.L. was admitted because her feeding tube had become dislodged, E.L. insisted upon immediate insertion of a central line and hyperalimentation. E.L. asserted that to do anything short of that would be tantamount to allowing her mother to starve to death. S.A. refused to consent to insertion of a central line and requested comfort measures only. These conflicting instructions exposed J.L.'s physicians to a battery claim if they inserted a central line (contrary to S.A.'s instructions) or a claim of negligence if they withheld inserting the central line (contrary to E.L.'s instructions).

E.L. retained an attorney within 24 hours of J.L.'s feeding tube becoming dislodged and filed an emergency petition for injunctive relief in the county court asking that the court order her mother's physicians to insert a central line and begin hyperalimentation. The court entered the order as requested.

At her final admission to our facility, J.L.'s treating physicians diagnosed her with renal failure, possible bowel ischemia, sepsis, and gastrointestinal bleeding. E.L. instructed the treating physicians to proceed with an exploratory laparotomy and dialysis. S.A., on the other hand, would not consent to either procedure. The attending surgeon acknowledged that the patient stood less than a 1 percent chance of surviving the surgery. Nevertheless, the surgeon was willing to perform the surgery because he feared being sued. Likewise, dialysis posed a serious risk because J.L. was already dangerously hypotensive and dialysis would lower her blood pressure even more. Notwithstanding the high risks of surgery and dialysis, E.L. insisted that both procedures be performed since her mother would certainly die without the interventions.

Once again E.L. retained counsel who filed another emergency petition with the local court asking the court to order the hospital to "undertake any medical or other care that is necessary to try and preserve the life [of J.L.]." Although the court declined to order surgery because to do so would almost certainly result in the patient's death, the court did order dialysis and "full resuscitation." Less than a week after the court entered its order, J.L. went into cardiac arrest. In accordance with the court order and E.L.'s wishes, physicians administered cardiopulmonary resuscitation for forty-five minutes without success.

Although a futility policy would not have avoided any of the litigation in this case, it would have afforded the treating physicians a venue in which to present the facts of their patient's medical condition and the likely outcome of the treatment requested by her daughter, E.L. Assuming the review board—known as the Institutional Interdisciplinary Review Board—had concluded that the laparotomy and dialysis were futile, J.L.'s physicians at least would then have had the endorsement of their own health care system if they had decided to forego treatment.[15] Perhaps the judge in this case would have ruled differently had the hospital been able to introduce into evidence the fact that J.L.'s case had been reviewed by both the Institutional Ethics Committee and the Institutional Interdisciplinary Review Board and that both had determined that the surgery and dialysis were medically futile treatments.

Futile-treatment decisions today incorporate medical, ethical, social, and legal components. The heart of the debate centers on the conflict between individual rights (patient autonomy) and the allocation of medical resources (social justice), but a central component of this debate must be what the physician believes is in the best interest of the patient. Absent statutory or appellate authority on futile treatment, physicians will have to balance the threat of litigation against their professional integrity in determining whether they can administer treatments that run counter to their professional judgment. This balancing act is dangerous because patients' lives hang in the balance. Futile-treatment policies will not only benefit physicians legally by confirming that the standard of care was not breached, it will also be in the best interest of patients and society as a whole.

ETHICAL ANALYSIS

Futility is defined as "inadequacy to produce a result or bring about a required end; ineffectiveness."[16] Medically, the concept of futility, according to the American Medical Association, "cannot be meaningfully defined."[17] Essentially, futility is a subjective judgment, but one that is realistically indispensable.[18] There is consensus within the medical community that, at specific times during the course of an illness, some treatments are medically futile. Consensus ends, however, when attempts are made to formulate a fully objective and concrete definition.

As a result, "futile treatment" became confused with interventions that are harmful, impossible, and ineffective. Distinguishing among these interventions has led to some clarity. In general, a medically futile treatment is "an action, intervention, or procedure that might be physiologically effective in a given case, but cannot benefit the patient, no matter how often it is repeated. A futile treatment is not necessarily ineffective, but it is worthless, either because the medical action itself is futile (no matter what the patient's condition) or the condition of the patient makes it futile."[19] But until we have a clearer understanding of what medical futility means at the bedside, there will not be widespread agreement on definitions and implications of futility in general.[20]

Ethicists Baruch Brody and Amir Halevy have distinguished four categories of medical futility that set the parameters for this debate. First, physiological futility, also known as quantitative futility, applies to treatments that fail to achieve their intended physiological effect. These determinations are based not on vague clinical impressions but on substantial information about the outcomes of specific interventions for different categories of patients. The second category, imminent-demise futility, refers to those instances in which, despite the proposed intervention, the patient will die in the very near future (this is sometimes expressed as the patient will not survive to discharge, although that is not really equivalent to dying in the very near future). Brody and Halevy use the third category, lethal-condition futility, to describe those cases in which the patient has an underlying lethal condition which the intervention does not affect and which will result in death in the not too distant future (weeks, perhaps months, but not years) even if the intervention is employed. The fourth category, qualitative futility, refers to instances in which an intervention fails to lead to an acceptable quality of life for the patient.[21] When a treatment is judged to be qualitatively futile, the claim being made is that, although the treatment may succeed in achieving an effect, the effect is not worth achieving from the patient's perspective.[22]

Medically, a consensus concerning the clinical features of medical futility remains elusive. "Whatever futility means, it seems obvious that this is not a discrete clinical concept with a sharp demarcation between futile and nonfutile treatment."[23] Brody and Halevy's four categories emphasize that decisions on medical futility must be made on a case-by-case basis and must include both a substantive component and a role for patient and surrogate input. Determining whether a medical treatment is futile basically comes down to deciding whether it passes the test of beneficence, that is, will this treatment be in the patient's "best interest." The test of beneficence is complex because determining whether a medical treatment is beneficial or burdensome, proportionate or disproportionate, appropriate or inappropriate, involves value judgments by both the patient and the physician.

Patients have the right of self-determination to control their own medical treatment, but this does not give patients the absolute right to demand any medical treatment. Physicians have the duty to practice medicine responsibly, that is, they are called to follow professional norms, standards, and values as guides to their judgments on the appropriateness of medical interventions for their patients. Of course, this does not mean that they can determine medical treatments for patients unilaterally.

Ethically, the issue of medical futility focuses on the conflict between the values of the patient and surrogate and the values of the physician. Medical judgments are never value-free. In determining whether a treatment is medically futile, physicians must consider carefully not only the values and goals of the patient and surrogate, they must also consider community and institutional standards. The values of the patient, physician, and society as a whole, are all part of this decision-making process. The question is this: How does the physician balance all these values so that the best interest of the patient is always the central focus? One can argue that the ethical principles of autonomy, beneficence, and justice will provide a moral framework, based on moral tradition, for making these medical and ethical decisions.

Autonomy refers to the right of a person to exercise self-determination in making personal and informed choices. In the case of medical futility, autonomy refers to the right of a patient or surrogate to choose from among certain medically justifiable options. The patient has the right to choose and refuse medical treatments, but the physician also has the right to make choices based on his or her duty to practice medicine responsibly. In this situation, both patient and physician have the right of autonomy in making these medical decisions. Legally and ethically, patients have been given the right to refuse medical treatments, but this right does not imply that they also have the right of access to any medical treatment. Patients have the right to make medical decisions they believe are in their best interest, but at times, due to various factors, these decisions may be destructive and irrational choices. It is at this point that patient autonomy conflicts with physician beneficence.

Physicians cannot be forced to make a decision concerning a medical treatment which they believe is not in the best interest of the patient or society as a whole. To do so would violate the professional norms of the physician—in that the physician would be asked to practice irrational medicine. To initiate or continue medical interventions even though the patient is no longer able to appreciate any benefit from these interventions is to confuse means with ends, effects with benefits, and available technologies with obligatory medical therapies.[24] This is not simply an irrational act, it is morally irresponsible.

The Christian view of autonomy focuses on the dignity and respect of every person. This does not mean that each and every person has absolute autonomy. "Respect for persons embraces self-governing decision making. But our freedom as creatures of God is always within the constraints of ethical and moral determinants derived from Scripture, tradition, Church teaching, and the study of ethics."[25] Therefore, to allow patients or surrogates to think that certain medical treatments are acceptable when they are futile is to mislead them. This violates the principle of autonomy in that "it creates a sphere of decision making where (rationally) none exists and, thus, seems intrinsically deceptive."[26] If the conflict between patient and physician prevents a consensus decision, then the only option for the patient is to terminate the patient–physician relationship and seek another physician. For the physician, there are three options: the physician can arrange for transfer of the patient, seek a declaratory judgment in court, or act without the patient's approval. Litigation may ensue with the last option, but if the physician has acted within generally accepted medical standards and/or in conformance with the expressed wishes of the patient, the physician should prevail.[27]

Beneficence involves the obligation to prevent and remove harms and to promote the good of the person by minimizing the burdens incurred and maximizing the benefits to the patient and others. Beneficence includes nonmaleficence, which prohibits inflicting harm, injury, or death upon others. In determining whether a particular treatment is beneficial to the patient, it is important to distinguish between quantitative futility and qualitative futility.

Quantitative futility is an objective assessment of a particular medical treatment that should be made by the physician. Schneiderman et al. have proposed that for a treatment to be medically futile it has to have been useless in the last one hundred cases of a physician's personal experience or in published reports. A treatment that merely preserves permanent unconsciousness or cannot end dependence on critical care should also be considered futile. Furthermore, in judging futility, physicians must distinguish between an effect, which is limited to a part of the patient's body, and a benefit, which appreciably improves the person as a whole.[28] Physicians have an ethical responsibility to provide those treatments to their patients which they believe will benefit them as a person and not harm them or be too burdensome for them. To directly harm a patient violates a basic tenet in the Hippocratic Oath—above all, do no harm—and violates the Christian notion of beneficence which means doing good out of love for the person in need.[29] Nevertheless, in determining whether a particular treatment is beneficial or nonbeneficial, patients and surrogates must also be permitted to determine the impact of that treatment on their quality of life.

In general, patients will make decisions that are rational and in their best interest, but situations arise when they may not be thinking rationally. "Commitment to beneficence demands at least that physicians try to understand patients' intent and motivation and to influence them to make a rational decision. In some cases, physicians may choose not to act on patient decisions that appear to be unreasonably destructive."[30] For a patient, discerning whether a medical treatment is beneficial or nonbeneficial is subjective and relies on the patient's assessment of his or her own good. This is a value judgment about what the patient (or surrogate) believes is in his or her best interests. Physicians need to take the time to communicate with their patients in order to better understand the physical, emotional, spiritual, and financial values that govern their lives. The values and goals of the patient should help to inform a physician's decisions, but they must be considered alongside the professional standards that reflect medical values and guide judgments about the appropriateness of a medical treatment.

Physicians have the expertise to determine whether a medical treatment is quantitatively futile. They should never comply with a patient's or surrogate's request to offer a treatment that is clearly physiologically futile, burdensome, and is certain only to prolong a seemingly meaningless life. Patients and surrogates are in the best position to determine whether a medical treatment is qualitatively futile, that is, beneficial or burdensome according to his or her values. Ideally, the physician and patient or surrogate together should come to a decision about the appropriateness of a particular medical treatment and whether such treatment will maximize the benefits and minimize the burdens for the patient. Shared decision making that is rooted in the concept of reasonableness and allows for flexibility, openness, and honesty is the only model that will pass the test of beneficence. Extreme medical paternalism and extreme patient autonomy not only fail the test of beneficence, but also may, at times, also fail the test of nonmaleficence.

The principle of justice recognizes that all people should be treated fairly and be given what they are due. The issue of medical futility focuses specifically on distributive justice, that is, the fair, equitable, and appropriate distribution of medical resources in society. In determining if a particular medical treatment is futile, one cannot ignore the question of social justice. At a time when health care reform is a priority in this country, proceeding with medical treatments that are judged to be futile and inappropriate is inconsistent with the standards of society and violates the principle of distributive justice. Access to basic health care benefits for all Americans might never be realized if we continue to offer unreasonable medical care.

Despite the important role distributive justice plays in the futility debate, it is rarely mentioned as a major factor. Mentioning cost factors and scarce resources in discerning the nonmaleficence of specific medical treatments brings the criticism that one is "putting a price tag on human life." To many Americans, this is totally unacceptable. "Human life is too important to assign a price to it." But is this realistic? Medical resources in this country and in the world are limited and must be conserved for just distribution. Proper stewardship of these medical resources entails not wasting them on medical treatments that are futile and inappropriate. Instead, these resources must be rationally allocated. To waste such resources when they are in short supply is both ethically irresponsible and morally objectionable.

Critics will argue that incorporating distributive justice into the medical futility debate is just a devious disguise for "medical rationing." This charge only confuses the issue. Futility judgments and allocation decisions are very different from rationing. Futility refers to specific treatments and outcome relationships with a specific patient. Rationing refers to withholding of efficacious treatments in the general population on a cost basis because of competing needs.[31] "Therefore, in making judgments about futility, the patient's benefit is of paramount concern, and all that matters is medicine's ability to offer some minimal promise to achieve that benefit. All other factors are extraneous. With respect to rationing, by contrast, society must decide how to deal with conditions of scarcity in which certain treatments cannot be made available to all who would benefit."[32]

As a matter of justice, patients and surrogates cannot be given the absolute right to demand any medical treatment. To do so would create a system that "would irrationally allocate health care to socially powerful people with strong preferences for immediate treatment to the disadvantage of those with less power and less immediate needs."[33] If patients and surrogates are given the absolute right to demand inappropriate and nonbeneficial medical treatments, this would be accomplished at the expense of the poor, the powerless, and the marginalized. Failure to consider the allocation of scarce resources in this debate would be a grave injustice.

The medical futility debate comes down to a conflict of patient autonomy versus physician beneficence and distributive justice. In seeking a balance between the values and goals of medicine and the values and goals of the patient, individual autonomy cannot be so inflated in importance as to destroy the principle of beneficence and overlook the equitable distribution of medical resources in society. To find this balance, physicians must reach a consensus on what constitutes a reasonable medical treatment, and patients and surrogates must restrict their self-advocacy to what is fair and equitable for all.[34] The focus of this debate must center on the best interest of the patient, without failing to recognize that every individual is also a member of society. If a physician believes, after carefully considering the patient's medical status, values, and goals, that a particular medical treatment is futile because it violates the principles of beneficence and justice, then the physician is ethically and professionally obligated to resist administering that treatment. The justification of medical treatments on the basis of weighing the benefits and burdens and the appropriate use of medical resources is firmly rooted in the Catholic moral tradition of distinguishing between ordinary and extraordinary means.

The Catholic tradition maintains that if a medical intervention is judged to be ordinary it is viewed as morally mandatory. If extraordinary, it is morally optional. It is said to be ordinary if it offers a reasonable hope of benefit for the patient and could be used without excessive inconvenience—which includes risk, pain, and expense. If it offers no reasonable hope or benefit or is excessively burdensome, it is extraordinary.[35] Pius XII further clarified the distinction when he declared that "we are morally obliged to use only ordinary means to preserve life and health—according to circumstances of persons, places, times, and culture—that is to say means that do not involve any grave burden for oneself or another."[36]

Pius XII based the distinction between ordinary and extraordinary means on the idea that human life is a basic good, but a good to be preserved precisely as a condition of other values. One must examine the circumstances of a particular situation, which includes cost factors and allocation of resources, because these circumstances dictate the balance to be considered between life and these other values. Due to the imprecision of the terms *ordinary means* and *extraordinary means* and the rapid advances in medicine and technology, the Catholic Church now speaks of *proportionate* and *disproportionate* means.

In determining if a medical treatment is beneficial and appropriate, the Congregation for the Doctrine of the Faith in the *Declaration on Euthanasia* concludes, "It will be possible to make a correct judgment as to the means by studying the type of treatment being used, its degree of complexity or risk, its cost and possibilities of using it, and comparing these elements with the result that can be expected, taking into account the state of the sick person and his or her physical and moral resources."[37] This statement, which is rooted in the Catholic tradition, gives physicians the ethical justification to refuse medical treatments if they are either gravely burdensome or medically futile for the patient.

After being confronted with the J.L. case, and other similar cases when surrogates and family members demanded medical treatments which were clearly futile (yet physicians capitulated), our Catholic Health System decided to formulate a medical futility policy that would address these concerns. Various types of futility policies were examined, and after careful review, it was determined that since there was no consensus on a substantive definition of futility, then a process-based approach for determining futility on a case-by-case basis was more appropriate. We based our policy on the Houston process-based approach because it seemed to be the most practical to implement.[38] After countless meetings, we designed a similar procedural policy that is firmly rooted in the Catholic tradition.

We also decided to dovetail this policy with a palliative care policy so that it would be very clear that, even though we may determine a specific treatment to be medically futile, we will never abandon a patient. Each patient will be given appropriate care and will be treated with the utmost dignity and respect. Catholic hospitals are called to embrace Christ's healing mission, which means to offer patients those treatments which will be beneficial to them. These treatments should restore their health, cure when possible, relieve pain and suffering, provide comfort, and improve their quality of life. The test of beneficence is whether or not physicians can achieve these goals, not just any goals or any interests.[39] A process-based futility policy will assist physicians in providing patients with medical treatments which are in their best interest, will foster a responsible stewardship of health care resources, and will provide the courts with a fair standard to be used in adjudicating these cases.

To help patients, surrogates, and health care providers better understand the concept of medical futility, Appendix A provides a copy of that futility policy, developed and used in a Catholic health care system. The basics of this policy, while grounded in the Catholic tradition, can serve as a model for a medical futility policy in any hospital. Appendix B is a copy of a neonatal/pediatric futility policy, designed while I was on sabbatical at the Center for Clinical Bioethics at Georgetown University Medical School. This policy was based on my experiences of working in the Neonatal Intensive Care Unit (NICU) at Georgetown University Hospital. Appendix C is a copy of a palliative care policy that should go hand in hand with any futility policy. These policies can serve as models to help resolve some of the questions regarding medical futility confronting patients, surrogates, physicians, and hospitals today.

APPENDIX A:
ADULT MEDICAL FUTILITY POLICY

PURPOSE:

This policy supplements existing policies on limiting life-prolonging therapies by providing a conflict-resolution mechanism to follow when a patient (or surrogate decision maker) requests an intervention that the attending physician assesses to be medically inappropriate.

POLICY:

In faithful imitation of Jesus Christ the healer, Catholic health care facilities have served the sick, the suffering, and the dying in various ways throughout history. This ministry of healing is rooted in the Christian belief that all people are created in the image and likeness of God (Genesis 1:26). Therefore, all human life is sacred and should be treated with dignity and respect from the moment of conception until death. Human life is a gift of God, but death is unavoidable. It is necessary therefore that we, without in anyway hastening the hour of death, should be able to accept it with full responsibility and dignity. It is true that death marks the end of our earthly existence, but at the same time it opens the door to eternal life. Therefore, all people must prepare themselves for this event in the light of human values, and Christians even more so in the light of faith.[1]

The task of medicine is to care even when we cannot cure. Physicians and their patients must continually evaluate the use of the technology at their disposal. Reflections on the innate dignity of human life in all its dimensions and on the purpose of medical care is indispensable for formulating a true moral judgment about the use of technology to maintain human life. The use of life-sustaining technology must be judged in light of the Christian meaning of life, suffering, and death.[2] Physicians, in imitation of Christ the healer, have the duty to make their skills available to all who are sick and dying, but they should never forget that it is more important to provide their patients with comfort, kindness, and charity. This service to the people of God is also a service to Christ, who said,

"As you did to one of the least of these my brethren, you did to me" (Matthew 25:40).

The traditional goals of medicine, like the goals of Catholic health care, have been to heal and to relieve suffering and pain. In recent years, the goal of respecting autonomous patient choices has motivated the establishment of policies that permit patients (or surrogate decision makers) to exercise that autonomy by refusing or limiting an unwanted intervention. These policies are limited to situations in which patients (or surrogate decision makers) refuse an intervention. This current policy, designed to supplement rather than to supplant currently existing policies on limiting life-prolonging therapies, provides a conflict-resolution mechanism to follow when a patient (or surrogate decision maker) requests, rather that refuses, an intervention that the attending physician of record assesses to be medically inappropriate (commonly referred to as medically futile).

This policy affirms both the traditional goals of medicine and the moral value of physician and institutional integrity in discerning the limits of medical interventions that are set forth in the "Ethical and Religious Directives for Catholic Health Care Services." Respect for this integrity provides the basis for the right to refuse to provide a medically inappropriate intervention. It complements the right of patient determination that must be given both voice and effect in any forum for medical decision making. This appeal to integrity is generally rooted in a combination of concerns such as avoiding harm to patients, avoiding provision of unseemly care, just allocation and good stewardship of medical resources, and the belief that human life is the basis of all good but is not itself an absolute good. This policy affirms the value of integrity so long as appropriate institutional review supports the determination of medical inappropriateness.

After following the procedures set forth in this policy, a medically inappropriate intervention may be withheld or withdrawn, without obtaining the agreement of the patient (or surrogate decision maker).

PROCEDURES:

> 1. When the attending of record determines that an intervention is medically inappropriate but the patient (or surrogate decision maker) insists that it be provided, the attending of record should discuss carefully with the patient (or surrogate decision maker) the nature of the ailment, the options (including palliative care and hospice care), the

prognosis, and the reasons why the interventions are medically inappropriate. The attending of record should explain that not providing the intervention in question does not mean abandoning appropriate medical care designed to promote comfort and dignity and humane care designed to provide emotional and spiritual support.

2. The attending of record should address with the patient (or surrogate decision maker) the options of transferring the patient to another physician or to another institution, or obtaining an independent medical opinion concerning the medical inappropriateness or medical futility of the intervention in question. The attending of record should also provide the patient (or surrogate decision maker) with a copy of these guidelines.

3. The assistance of institutional resources (nursing staff, patient care representative, chaplain, and social services staff) must be made available to the patient (or the surrogate decision maker) and the attending of record.

4. If, after reasonable effort by the attending of record using the available institutional resources, agreement is not reached between the attending of record and the patient (or surrogate decision maker), the attending of record who still wishes to limit the intervention must request from the appropriate department director a second medical opinion from a physician who has personally examined the patient. The second opinion must be appropriately documented in the patient's chart. Within 48 hours of obtaining the second opinion, the attending of record must prepare the case for review and forward it to the Institutional Ethics Committee. The attending of record must provide to that body clinical and scientific information pertinent to the determination that the intervention is medically inappropriate. Within 48 hours after receipt of the case by the attending of record, the Institutional Ethics Committee must convene to hear the case. The attending of record and the patient (or surrogate decision maker) are requested to appear at the Institutional Ethics Committee meeting to represent their points of view. The Committee will render its recommendations no later than 24 hours after hearing the case. A representative of the Ethics Committee will meet with both parties together to review and discuss the recommendations of the Committee.

5. In the event that both parties cannot reach a consensus after receiv-

ing the recommendations of the Institutional Ethics Committee, all information will be forwarded by the Institutional Interdisciplinary Review Board (IIRB)[3] for adjudication.

6. The attending of record must notify the patient (or surrogate decision maker) in writing that the case has been forwarded to the IIRB, what it involves, what its possible outcomes are, when and where the review will take place, and that there is still the option of transferring before the meeting, but that arranging such a transfer is the responsibility of the patient (or surrogate decision maker). Absent patient (or surrogate decision maker) consent to an earlier time, the meeting cannot take place for at least forty-eight (48) hours after the patient (or surrogate decision maker) is notified.

7. During the IIRB process, the attending of record and the patient (or surrogate decision maker) are encouraged to be present together to express their views for consideration, including alternative plans of care. This meeting of the IIRB should occur at the acute-care facility where the patient is currently hospitalized to facilitate access to the patient and the patient's record's.

8. If a finding of medical inappropriateness is affirmed by the IIRB, medically inappropriate intervention may be terminated and a plan of care established that addresses comfort care and the preservation of patient dignity.[4] If, however, the IIRB does not concur with the attending of record's determination of medical inappropriateness, the orders to limit the intervention will not be recognized as valid without patient (or surrogate decision maker) agreement.

9. If the IIRB agrees with the determination of medical inappropriateness, intrainstitutional system transfers of the care of the patient to another physician to provide palliative care are allowed. However, intrainstitutional system transfers to another physician to provide the intervention that has been judged by the IIRB to be medically inappropriate will not be allowed.

10. The procedures set forth in this policy may be invoked only by the attending of record or as otherwise authorized by the hospital's medical staff by-laws. Concerns on the part of other health care providers, hospital officials, or family members should be addressed through already existing institutional mechanisms.

RESPONSIBILITY:

Hospital Administration at each facility is responsible for the effective implementation of this policy.

Notes

[1] Sacred Congregation for the Doctrine of the Faith, *Declaration on Euthanasia*, 1980.

[2] United States Conference of Catholic Bishops, "Ethical and Religious Directives for Catholic Health Care Services" 1995, part 5.

[3] The Institutional Interdisciplinary Review Board will be a Health Care System Review Board that will be in acute-care facilities within the system. The Board members will consist of a physician, a nurse, a social worker, a representative of mission services, a pastoral care member, the bioethicist, and legal counsel. The Board will be appointed annually by the Senior Vice-President for Mission and Sponsorship.

[4] Refer to the Palliative Care Policy.

APPENDIX B:
PROPOSED POLICY ON THE DETERMINATION OF MEDICALLY INAPPROPRIATE MEDICAL TREATMENT FOR PEDIATRIC AND NEONATAL CENTERS

PURPOSE AND POLICY:

The traditional goals of medicine have been to heal and to relieve suffering and pain. The specific task of medicine is to care even when we cannot cure. As a result, physicians and their patients/surrogates must continually evaluate the use of technology at their disposal. Reflections on the innate dignity of human life in all its dimensions and on the purpose of medical care is indispensable for formulating a true moral judgment about the use of technology to maintain human life. In recent years, the goal of respecting autonomous patient choices has motivated the establishment of policies that permit patients/surrogates to exercise that autonomy by refusing or limiting an unwanted intervention. These policies are limited to situations in which patients/surrogates refuse an intervention. This current policy, designed to supplement rather than to supplant currently existing policies on limiting life-prolonging therapies, provides a conflict-resolution mechanism to follow when a patient/surrogate requests, rather than refuses, an intervention that the attending physician of record assesses to be medically inappropriate (commonly referred to as medically futile).

This policy affirms both the traditional goals of medicine and the moral value of physician and institutional integrity in discerning the limits of medical interventions. Respect for this integrity provides the basis for the right to refuse to provide a medically inappropriate intervention. It complements the right of patient determination that must be given both voice and effect in any forum for medical decision making. This appeal to integrity is generally rooted in a combination of concerns such as avoiding harm to patients, avoiding provision of unseemly care, just allocation and good stewardship of medical resources, and the belief that human life is the basis of all goods but is not itself an absolute good. This policy affirms the value of integrity so long as appropriate institutional review supports the determination of medical inappropriateness.

61

It should be noted that in most cases the decision maker will be the parent(s) of the child, except in those instances where the child is an emancipated or mature minor. However, when developmentally appropriate, especially with older children and adolescents, physicians should also solicit a patient assent from these children. [American Academy of Pediatrics, "Informed Consent, Parental Permission, and Assent in Pediatric Practice," *Pediatrics* (February 1995): 1–7.]

After following the procedures set forth in this policy, a medically inappropriate intervention may be withheld or withdrawn without obtaining the agreement of the patient/surrogate.

PROCEDURES:

1. When the attending of record determines that an intervention is medically inappropriate but the patient/surrogate insists that it be provided, the attending of record should discuss carefully with the patient/surrogate the nature of the ailment, the options (including palliative care and hospice care), the prognosis, and the reasons why the interventions are medically inappropriate. [Treatments are inappropriate when they provide no reasonable possibility of extended life or other benefit to the patient, and treatments are harmful when additional suffering or other harm inflicted is grossly disproportionate to any possibility of benefit. These definitions are adopted from T. Tomlinson and D. Czlonka, "Futility and Hospital Policy," *Hastings Center Report* 95 (1995): 28–35.] The attending of record should explain that not providing the intervention in question does not mean abandoning appropriate medical care designed to promote comfort and dignity and humane care designed to provide emotional and spiritual support.

2. The attending of record should address with the patient/surrogate the options of transferring the patient to another physician or to another institution, or obtaining an independent medical opinion concerning the medical inappropriateness or medical futility of the intervention in question. The attending of record should also provide the patient/surrogate with a copy of these guidelines.

3. The assistance of institutional resources (nursing staff, patient care representative, chaplain, and social services staff) shall be made available to the patient/surrogate and to the attending of record.

4. If, after reasonable effort by the attending of record using the available institutional resources, agreement is not reached between the attending of record and the patient/surrogate, the attending of record who still wishes to limit the intervention must request from the Department Director a second medical opinion from a physician, preferably from another institution, who has personally examined the patient. The second opinion must be appropriately documented in the patient's chart. Within 48 hours of obtaining the second opinion, the attending of record must prepare the case for review and forward it to the Institutional Ethics Committee. The attending of record must provide to that body clinical and scientific information pertinent to the determination that the intervention is medically inappropriate.

5. Within 48 hours after receipt of the case by the attending of record, the Institutional Ethics Committee must convene to hear the case. The attending of record and the patient/surrogate are requested to appear at the Institutional Ethics Committee meeting to represent their points of view. The Committee will render its recommendations no later than 24 hours after hearing the case. A representative of the Institutional Ethics Committee will meet with both parties together to review and discuss the recommendations of the Committee.

6. In the event that both parties cannot reach a consensus after receiving the recommendation of the Institutional Ethics Committee, all information will be forwarded by the Institutional Ethics Committee to the Pediatric Treatment Review Board (PTRB) for adjudication. [The PTRB will consist of a pediatrician, neonatologist, nurse, social worker, pastoral care member, psychiatrist/psychologist, bioethicist, legal counsel, and a hospital administrator. The Chairperson of the Board will be selected by the Board members prior to the meeting. The Board will be appointed yearly by the Senior Vice-President for Medical Affairs for the hospital/system. In addition, the Senior Vice-President for Medical Affairs will also appoint *ex officio* a physician from each specialty to serve as a consultant to the PTRB when appropriate. Efforts should be made to attain ethnic and cultural diversity, in order to represent the variety of experiences of health and illness among different groups.]

7. The attending of record must notify the patient/surrogate in writing that the case has been forwarded to the PTRB, what it involves, what its possible outcomes are, when and where the review will take place,

and that there is still the option of transferring before the meeting, but that arranging such a transfer is the responsibility of the patient/surrogate. Absent patient/surrogate consent to an earlier time, the meeting cannot take place for at least forty-eight (48) hours after the patient/surrogate is notified. The patient/surrogate should feel free to bring legal counsel, if desired, and the hospital should provide reasonable assistance in this regard, if requested by the patient/surrogate. However, it should be made clear to all parties that this is not a legal proceeding.

8.   During the PTRB process, the attending of record and the patient/surrogate are encouraged to be present together to express their views for consideration—including alternative plans of care. Board members should have ample opportunity to ask questions about the case so that everyone present has an adequate understanding of the relevant issues. The purpose of the questions should be to seek to understand the differences in values and interpretation of the facts that have led to the conflict. As much as possible, the Board should strive to attain the perspective of the patient/surrogate in an effort to grasp the essential differences that exist between them and the clinicians.

Some patients/surrogates may refuse to meet with the PTRB. This may be a reflection of the loss of trust that has developed between the clinician and the patient and family in the process. Nevertheless, when good faith efforts have been made to include the patient/surrogate/family in the process, then their refusal to meet with the Board should neither be seen as undermining the integrity of the process nor invalidating the Board's recommendations. This meeting of the PTRB should occur at the acute-care facility where the patient is currently hospitalized to facilitate access to the patient and the patient's records.

9. If a finding of medical inappropriateness is affirmed by the PTRB, medically inappropriate intervention may be terminated and a plan of care established that addresses comfort care and the preservation of patient dignity. [This refers to the hospital's Palliative Care Policy.] If, however, the PTRB does not concur with the attending of record's determination of medical inappropriateness, the orders to limit the intervention will not be recognized as valid without patient/surrogate agreement.

10. If the PTRB agrees with the determination of medical inappropriateness, intrainstitutional system transfers of the care of the patient

to another physician to provide palliative care are allowed. However, intrainstitutional system transfers to another physician to provide the intervention that has been judged by the PTRB to be medically inappropriate will not be allowed. Permission should be sought to transfer the patient to another facility. If this fails, possible options are not well-defined. On the one hand, physicians have a moral obligation not to abandon patients under their care, while on the other hand, medical professionals should not be obligated to provide treatments in violation of their clinical judgments, consciences, and ethical standards. This direction therefore does not provide specific recommendations for this possible outcome.

11. The procedures set forth in this policy may be invoked only by the attending of record or as otherwise authorized by the hospital's medical staff by-laws. Concerns on the part of other health care providers, hospital officials, or family members should be addressed through already existing institutional mechanisms.

Appendix C:
Adult Palliative Care: Policy and Procedure

Purpose:

The purposes of this policy are to:
- Clarify the meaning of palliative care, often referred to as "comfort care."
- Promote comprehensive and consistent palliative care.
- Establish a process of determining appropriate palliative care for individual patients.

Policy:

The Health System recognized that in the care of patients with advanced disease it is medically appropriate and ethically acceptable to shift the primary goal of treatment of palliative care if this is judged to be medically appropriate by the patient's physician and consistent with the wishes of the patient or the patient's surrogate.

I. Definition:

Palliative care consists of all treatments and services aimed at alleviating physical symptoms and addressing the psychological, social, and spiritual needs of the patients and their families so as to enhance patients' and families' quality of life to the greatest degree possible.

Palliative Care

- affirms life and regards dying as a normal process;
- implies the cessation of all diagnostic measures and all life-sustaining and other therapeutic treatments that do not directly contribute to the patient's comfort or to patient and family goals; and

- consists of active management of pain and other distressing symptoms. In the relief of pain, it is ethically permissible to administer analgesics in sufficient amounts to control the patient's pain—even if this has the unintended effect of depressing the patient's respiratory function.

II. Procedure:

A. A discussion should be initiated between the attending physician and the patient and /or the patient's family about the appropriateness of shifting goals of treatment to palliative care.

B. The attending physician and other members of the health care team should develop a palliative care plan with the patient's family (usually in the context of a family conference), taking into account their particular goals and needs. Special attention should be given to:

- what therapies and procedures should be continued, discontinued, or initiated;
- symptom control, especially the management of pain and anxiety;
- the most appropriate setting for the patient's death to occur, including the appropriateness of hospice care.

C. The physician should document the patient's and/or family's agreement with the plan in the medical record.

D. The physician should complete the "Palliative Care Order Form." A general order—"comfort care only"—is not acceptable.

E. A regular review of the palliative care plan should occur and adjustments should be made as the patient's condition changes.

Adult Palliative Care Order Form

Date: _____

Time: _____

1.   Resuscitation status

This patient is no-CPR. In the event of cardiac or respiratory arrest, cardiopulmonary resuscitation will not be attempted. No "code blue" should be called.

2.   Initiate the following orders to provide comfort:

Pain/air hunger: _____

Anxiety/delirium: _____

Sleep: _____

Constipation: _____

Diarrhea: _____

Nausea/vomiting: _____

Thirst: _____

Fever: _____

Other: _____

3.   The following therapies might not contribute to providing comfort. If this patient is currently receiving any of these, please indicate below if they are to be continued or discontinued.

IV hydration	Continue	Discontinue
Diagnostic procedures	Continue	Discontinue
ECG and O2 sat monitoring	Continue	Discontinue
Supplemental O2	Continue	Discontinue
Parenteral and/or		
Enteral nutrition	Continue	Discontinue
Arterial lines	Continue	Discontinue
Central venous lines	Continue	Discontinue
Peripheral venous lines	Continue	Discontinue
PT/OT	Continue	Discontinue
Blood products	Continue	Discontinue
Radiation therapy	Continue	Discontinue
Dialysis (Please notify nephrologist, Dr. _____)		
	Continue	Discontinue
Blood draws for standing laboratory orders		
	Continue	Discontinue

4.   Please discontinue the following medications: _____

_____

5.   Consult Pastoral Care and Social Work Departments.

6.   Hospice Department to evaluate patient appropriateness of hospice care.

Transfer Orders: _____

_____

FOUR:
"DO NOT RESUSCITATE" ORDERS, ADVANCE DIRECTIVES/LIVING WILLS, AND DURABLE POWERS OF ATTORNEY FOR HEALTH CARE

In the year 1900, there were 3.1 million Americans over the age of 65 (or 4.1 percent of the population). By mid-century, there were 12.3 million people over 65 (or 8.1 percent of the population). In 2000, 35.0 million people were over 65 (or 12.4 percent of the population), a number that is projected to rise to 71.5 million by 2030 (or 19.6 percent of the population) when the youngest baby-boomers will have passed age 65. . . . In 1900, the usual place of death was at home; in 2000, it was the hospital. In 1900, most people died from accidents or infections without suffering a long period of disability. In 2000, people suffered, on average, two years of severe disability on the way to death. Acute causes of death (such as pneumonia, influenza, and septicemia) are in decline; prolonged causes of death from age-related degenerative diseases (such as Alzheimer's, Parkinson's, and emphysema) are on the rise.[1]

Joanne Lynn, who has studied disability and aging in America argues, "Most Americans die with failure of a major organ (heart, lungs, kidneys, or liver), dementia, stroke, or general frailty of old age. . . . These conditions lead to long periods of diminished function and involve multiple unpredictable and serious exacerbations of symptoms."[2] As a result, questions have arisen about the appropriateness of certain aggressive medical treatments during these prolonged periods of disability. Do patients want aggressive medical treatment when they have an end-stage medical condition? Are these treatments in the best interest of the patient? Do we know the wishes of patients regarding end-of-life treatment? Finally, are physicians and family members abiding by the wishes of patients regarding end-of life medical treatment?

"In the last three decades of the twentieth century, a series of court cases—Karen Ann Quinlan (1976), Brother Fox (1979), Claire Conroy

(1985), Nancy Cruzan (1990), and Nancy B (Canada, 1992) among them—attempted to deal with these questions. Invariably, self-determination was affirmed. The individual patient or the patient's surrogate is the ultimate decision maker concerning possible treatment options."[3] Since the 1990s, however, with advancements in medicine and technology, medical decision making has become even more complex. In 2006, Pennsylvania Governor Edward Rendell's Task Force for Quality at the End of Life issued a report, "Improving End-of-Life Experiences for Pennsylvanians," that urged more support to family caregivers, better education and higher standards for health professionals, and improved, more supportive policies governing advance directives and greater awareness of advance care planning through education of health care professionals and the broader community.[4]

What has become evident is that the process of aging and even dying has changed greatly over the last two decades due to advancements in medicine and technology, but the health care system and health care professionals have not kept pace with these changes. "The price of longer lives is longer, slower deaths. People rarely die quickly anymore. They decline and live years with debilitating, isolating incurable diseases."[5] Honoring the wishes of patients at the end of life has become problematic because in many instances family members and primary-care physicians do not know what the patient would want when confronted with these end-of-life situations. Conversations about end-of-life treatments are not taking place between patient and physician or between patient and families because we live in a "death-denying culture."

We hide from death, attempt to ignore death, and are even so arrogant as to think we can conquer death. It has become quite evident that Americans are still uncomfortable and even unrealistic about death and dying. There is a need to develop a systematic way that these vital conversations can be initiated so that when treatment decisions need to be made at the end of life and the patient is no longer competent, both the primary-care physician and the family know the values and wishes of the patient and are willing to carry them out.

Three documents in particular can assist patients, family members, and physicians in both the initiation of a conversation about end-of-life treatment and care and the fulfillment of a person's wishes. These documents can also serve to assure patients that, when a cure is no longer possible, they will die in comfort—with dignity and respect. This chapter will discuss "do not resuscitate" (DNR) orders, advance directives/living wills, and durable powers of attorney for health care. These documents are often misunderstood or confused with one another, and are often never discussed, initiated, or followed. Here, each document will be explained, discussed, and analyzed, and representative samples of each document will be provided.

Do Not Resuscitate (DNR) Orders:

It is estimated that every year in the United States more than a million people suffer cardiac arrest. About half of these people (515,000) die as a result. More than 250,000 of these coronary heart disease deaths occur without the victim ever reaching the hospital.[6] Cardiopulmonary resuscitation (CPR) is a specific set of medical procedures designed to establish circulation and breathing in a patient who has suffered an arrest of both. CPR is a supportive therapy, designed to maintain perfusion of vital organs while attempts are made to restore spontaneous breathing and cardiac rhythm.[7] CPR may involve simple efforts such as mouth-to-mouth resuscitation and external chest compressions or advanced efforts such as electric shock, insertion of a tube to open the patient's airway, injection of medications directly into the heart—and, in extreme cases, open chest massage. It should be made clear that CPR is a temporary procedure that can be used to maintain some blood flow to the brain, heart, and other vital organs until trained medical personnel are available to provide more advanced treatment.

"Studies have found that CPR is most effective when trained medical personnel arrive within 8 to 12 minutes of the arrest. Cardiopulmonary resuscitation should be performed only by persons trained in the technique because specific CPR recommendations vary depending on the patient's age and the cause of the arrest."[8] The problem is that two studies have found that even well-trained providers do not perform CPR according to the guidelines set forth by the American Heart Association and the International Liaison Committee on Resuscitation.[9]

Even though the public has the perception that CPR is quite effective, mainly because of television shows like "ER" and "Grey's Anatomy," the survival rates remain relatively low. "Despite decades of efforts to promote CPR science and education, the survival rate for out-of-hospital cardiac arrest remains low worldwide, averaging 6 percent or less."[10] Of those taken to the hospital with a cardiac arrest, it is estimated that the likelihood of surviving to leave the hospital ranges from 2 percent to 30 percent. For the average elderly person, this number hovers around 5 percent according to medical literature. Hospitalized patients who suffer cardiac arrest fare even worse, as these patients are usually sicker—with other comorbidities. Only an estimated 2 percent to 15 percent survive to discharge.[11]

According to a Canadian study "survival following cardiopulmonary resuscitation in hospital does not appear to have changed markedly in forty years."[12] The basic problem is that when patients or surrogates are approached by a physician regarding "code status" (If you go into cardiac or respiratory arrest, do you wish to be resuscitated?), they oftentimes are not told the survival rate or even what a "code" would entail. This violates the patient's right of informed consent.

Any patient who does not wish to undergo lifesaving treatment in the event of cardiac or respiratory arrest can request a "Do Not Resuscitate" order. The DNR order was first described in the United States in the 1960s when defibrillation allowed the reversal of cardiac arrest, but this might prolong the life of the patient for only a short time.[13] A DNR order is also referred to as the "code status" of a patient. A patient can be a "full code" when all life-sustaining measures will be attempted in the event that the patient goes into cardiac or respiratory arrest.

A patient can be a "no code" or what we refer to as having a DNR order written on his or her chart (see Appendixes A and B with this chapter). A DNR order, which is consented to by a patient or surrogate and written by a physician, is a physician's order that tells health care professionals that, if this particular patient suffers cardiopulmonary arrest, the patient should not be resuscitated. It should be noted that some states require one or two witnesses attesting to the fact that the patient is of sound mind, and under no duress, fraud, or undue influence.

Or a patient can be a "limited code," which means that only certain procedures will be done, such as allowing for chest compressions and antiarrhythmic drugs (to prevent or relieve cardiac arrhythmia), but no endotracheal intubation or mechanical ventilation will be performed (see Appendix C).[14] Limited codes, under most circumstances, are not medically appropriate. The problem is that if a person wants antiarrhythmic drugs but no chest compressions, then the drugs are injected but are not circulated and thus they give no benefit to the patient. Under most circumstances, "limited codes" are written because patients or surrogates fail to understand the full dimensions of a DNR order or fear the patient will be "abandoned."

There is also something called a "slow code" or what has been referred to as a "partial," "show," "light blue," or "Hollywood" code. This is when a patient is either a full code or a limited code and the medical professionals make a deliberate decision not to attempt aggressively to resuscitate. This is a half-hearted attempt where the full armamentarium of pharmacologic and mechanical interventions is not used, or where the length of the effort is shortened so that a full attempt at resuscitation is not made.[15] A "slow code" is unethical and illegal because it undermines the patient's right to self-determination and also violates the patient's trust in the medical professionals to abide by the agreed upon wishes of the patient or surrogate.

The confusion or lack of understanding surrounding code status is often due to the failure of physicians to explain DNR orders correctly. Unless patients or surrogates understand the full implications of what a "code status" entails, they cannot give informed consent. To give informed consent, the patient or surrogate should understand the survival rate, the trauma that is involved in a "code," and the quality of life that might result even if the code is successful. The patient or surrogate should also understand that a DNR order is only a decision about CPR and does not relate to other treatments.

Often even medical professionals misunderstand a DNR order to mean the foregoing of aggressive treatment in general. This is absolutely not the case. A patient can have a DNR order and still receive aggressive treatment for their medical condition. A patient can have a DNR order and still be in an intensive-care unit (ICU). Another problem associated with DRN orders is that the terminology "do not resuscitate" seems very harsh, cold, and even cruel. "Do Not Resuscitate" is often misunderstood by patients and surrogates as "do nothing"—the effective abandonment of the patient. To address this issue, a number of states are considering legislation to change the terminology in their relevant state codes from DNR to "Allow Natural Death" (AND) (See Appendix D). Georgia Health Decisions, a nonprofit, nonpartisan organization that works to promote public involvement in health issues is working with the Georgia legislature to make this change.[16]

Many might argue that using the terminology DNR or AND is basically a matter of semantics. This may be true, but when talking with a patient or family about code status, AND sounds "softer, more comforting, [and] warmer even though it contains a form of the 'D' word. It says that the team cares and will continue to care for the family member."[17] Basically what AND does is allow the physician to explain that in the event of a cardiac arrest the medical team will do everything possible to make the patient comfortable, but will allow the patient to die naturally and peacefully. This may seem like semantics, but we have found in practice that patients and family members react very positively to this terminology and it then allows the physician, when appropriate, to initiate a conversation about comfort measures, palliative care, and in some instances, even hospice care.

DNR orders are written for patients in a hospital setting, nursing home, or even in some states, for patients at home. To be valid, there may be a specific form that must be filled out with the signature of the physician and (in some cases) the patient or surrogate. The exact rules for obtaining and for emergency personnel accepting the validity of a DNR order vary widely according to jurisdiction. In many states, such as Pennsylvania, every time a patient moves from one institution (nursing home) to another (hospital) the DNR order must be rewritten to be valid. This is done to allow patients and surrogates the opportunity to reevaluate and even revise the code status when there is a change in the patient's medical condition.

The problem that often arises is that an unconscious patient is rushed to an Emergency Department in the middle of the night and it is hard to contact the patient's surrogate to confirm the code status. Consequently, the patient is a full code until the physician can obtain consent from the surrogate. Another example is when a terminal patient who is on home hospice with a DNR order goes into cardiac arrest and a family member becomes anxious and calls 911. The Emergency Medical Technicians (EMTs) or the paramedics arrive at the home, and if the person's heart or breathing has stopped, they will initiate treatment to restart the heart or breathing. To eliminate this problem, some states, like Pennsylvania, have adopted "Out-of-Hospital Do Not Resuscitate Orders."

On November 29, 2006, Pennsylvania enacted a statute (P.L. 1484, No. 169) that repealed the "DNR Act" and replaced it with the "Out-of-Hospital Nonresuscitation Act" (20 Pa. C.S. 5481–5488). The Act empowers a person who is competent and eighteen years of age or older with an end-stage medical condition (or an appropriate representative of that person) to secure an out-of-hospital DNR order and, at the person's option or the option of an authorized representative, an out-of-hospital DNR bracelet or necklace. These necklaces and bracelets can be obtained from the Pennsylvania Department of Health. The out-of-hospital DNR order is a written order that is issued by the person's attending physician that directs Emergency Medical Service (EMS) personnel to withhold CPR from the person in the event of the person's cardiac or respiratory arrest. The Act also specifies the circumstances under which an appropriate representative of the person who issued a living will under the "Living Will Act" (20 Pa. C.S. 5441–5447) is able to secure an out-of-hospital DRN order, bracelet or necklace for the person (see Appendix E).[18]

The effectiveness of a DNR order depends on the hospital in which the cardiopulmonary event occurs and the terms laid out in the specific DNR. If a patient has a DNR order, neither cardiopulmonary resuscitation nor intubation will be performed, but treatment for infections or other treatable conditions, intravenous feeding and fluids, and pain management and comfort care are generally continued. To violate a DNR order is both illegal and unethical because it violates the person's right to self-determination.

ADVANCE DIRECTIVES/LIVING WILLS

The origin of advance directives and living wills can be traced back to the beginnings of the euthanasia movement in the United States. "Some people wanted their written wishes, such as to be euthanized when they were no longer competent, to be legally binding. . . . The difficulty of making decisions for noncompetent patients, however, opened up the possibility of using a similar kind of document to guide treatment decisions, particularly at the end of life."[19] These documents became legal on November 5, 1990 when the United States Congress passed the "Federal Patient Self-Determination Act" (PSDA), which was an amendment to the "Omnibus Budget Reconciliation Act" of 1990. This act became effective on December 1, 1991.

The PSDA requires Medicare and Medicaid providers (hospitals, nursing homes, hospice programs, home health agencies, and HMOs) to give adult individuals, at the time of inpatient admission or enrollment, certain information about their rights under state laws governing advance directives—including the right to make decisions concerning medical care, the right to accept or refuse medical or surgical treatment, the right to formulate advance directives, and information on the provider's policies that govern the utilization of these rights. The act also prohibits institutions from discriminating against a patient who does not have an advance directive. This act further requires institutions to document patient information and provide ongoing community education on advance directives.[20] Even though polls show that patients and physicians strongly support advance directives and living wills, the medical literature consistently shows that only 15 to 20 percent of patients complete these forms. The other problem is that, of those completed, physicians often do not honor them and patients with advance directives or living wills receive no measurably different care at the end of life than patients without them.[21]

An advance directive is a document which indicates specific deci-

sions an individual would like made should he or she be unable to participate in the decision-making process. In some cases, this document may
spell out specific decisions, such as in a living will, while in others it may
designate a specific person to make health care decisions for the person.
In that case, the document is called a durable power of attorney for health
care—or it can be a combination document.[22]

A living will is a specific document that allows individuals to describe their wishes and values about the initiation or discontinuance of
death-delaying procedures in the event that they are incompetent and either
in a terminal, end-stage state or permanently unconscious (see Appendix
G). The durable power of attorney for health care is a specific document
that allows an individual (known as the principal) to appoint a particular
person (known as a surrogate or proxy)—or persons—to direct health care
decisions should the principal be unable to do so. This surrogate or proxy
should know the principal's values and wishes and have discussed what
the principal would want in the event he or she is terminally ill or in an
end-stage condition and is incompetent or permanently unconscious.

It should be noted that there are different types of powers of attorney (POAs). There have been situations in the hospital in which an individual identifies himself or herself as the POA for the patient and wants to
make medical decisions for that individual, but in reality they are the POA
only for financial matters. It is imperative that if someone identifies himself
or herself as the durable power of attorney for health care that this particular
individual produce the proper document with the necessary signatures appointing him or her to this position. This document should then be placed
on the patient's chart.

There is no universal, standard form for advance directives, living
wills, or durable power of attorney for health care. It is basically a written
form expressing the wishes of an individual regarding the initiation, continuation, withholding, or withdrawing of life-sustaining treatment and may
include other specific directions. Depending on the individual state, some
may need to be witnessed or in some cases notarized. Some states place a
time limit on the document, and some allow refusal of treatment resulting
in death only under certain circumstances.[23] Each of these is a legal document but, there is no need to have it written by legal counsel. Most state
legislatures have made the process citizen-friendly so that most adults can
easily write such a document. To assist individuals with these forms, the
U. S. Living Will Registry's website (http://www.uslivingwillregistry.com/
forms.shtm) lists links to each state so that individuals can download the
specific forms proposed by each of the 50 states.

Even though there are no universal forms for these documents, the requirements are rather standard in each state. The state of Pennsylvania recently passed a new law, Act 169 "Health Care Power of Attorney/Living Will Act" that went into effect January 29, 2007. Since this is a relatively new law governing advance directives, we will use it as the basis for information and discussion. (It should be noted that any advance directive written before January 29, 2007 continues to be valid in Pennsylvania provided it meets all the statutory requirements under the law now repealed—"Advance Directive for Health Care Act.")

Before discussing the requirements, it is important that we understand the terminology used in most state statutes regarding advance directives. The following are the definitions of the pertinent terms given in Pennsylvania Act 169:

> **advance health care directive:** A health care power of attorney, a living will, or a written combination of a health care power of attorney and living will.

> **attending physician:** The physician who has primary responsibility for the health care of a principal or patient.

> **competent:** A condition in which an individual, when provided appropriate medical information, communication supports, and technical assistance, is documented by a health care provider to do *all of the following*:
>
>> 1. Understand the potential material benefits, risks, and alternatives involved in a specific proposed health care decision.
>> 2. Make that health care decision on his or her own behalf.
>> 3. Communicate that health care decision to any other person.
>
> This term is intended to permit individuals to be found competent to make some health care decisions, but incompetent to make others.

> **end-stage medical condition:** An incurable and irreversible medical condition in an advanced state caused by injury, disease, or phys-

ical illness that will, in the opinion of the attending physician to a reasonable degree of medical certainty, result in death despite the introduction or continuation of medical treatment. Except as specifically set forth in an advance health care directive, the term is not intended to preclude treatment of a disease, illness, or physical, mental, cognitive, or intellectual condition, even if incurable and irreversible and regardless of severity, if *both* of the following apply:

1. The patient would benefit from the medical treatment, including palliative care.
2. Such treatment would not erely prolong the process of dying.

health care: Any care, treatment, service, or procedure to maintain, diagnose, treat, or provide for physical or mental health; and custodial or personal care, including any medication program, therapeutic and surgical procedure, and life-sustaining treatment.

health care agent: An individual designated by a principal in an advance health care directive.

health care decision: A decision regarding an individual's health care, including but not limited to the following:

1. Selection and discharge of a health care provider.
2. Approval or disapproval of a diagnostic test, surgical procedure, or program of medication.
3. Directions to initiate, continue, withhold, or withdraw all forms of life-sustaining treatment, including instructions not to resuscitate.

health care power of attorney: A writing made by a principal designating an individual to make health care decisions for the principal.

health care provider: A person who is licensed, certified, or otherwise authorized by the laws of the Commonwealth of Pennsylvania to administer or provide health care in the ordinary course of business or practice of a profession.

health care representative: An individual authorized under the Health Care Agents and Representatives Act to make health care decisions for a principal, provided that conditions set forth in section IV (b) (iii) of this policy have been met.

incompetent: A condition in which an individual, despite being provided appropriate medical information, communication supports, and technical assistance, is documented by a health care provider to be unable

1. to understand the potential material benefits, risks, and alternatives involved in a specific proposed health care decision; or
2. to make that health care decision on his or her own behalf; or
3. to communicate that health care decision to any other person.

The term is intended to permit individuals to be found incompetent to make some health care decisions, but competent to make others.

life-sustaining treatment: Any medical procedure or intervention that, when administered to a patient or principal who has an end-stage medical condition or is permanently unconscious, will serve only to prolong the process of dying or maintain the individual in a state of permanent unconsciousness. In the case of an individual with an Advance Directive, the term includes nutrition and hydration administered by gastric tube or intravenously or any other artificial or invasive means if the advance health care directive so specifically provides.

living will: A writing made in accordance with the Living Will Act that expresses a principal's wishes and instructions for health care and health care directions when the principal is determined to be incompetent and has an end-stage medical condition or is permanently unconscious.

permanently unconscious: A medical condition that has been diagnosed in accordance with currently accepted medical standards and with reasonable medical certainty as total and irreversible loss of consciousness and capacity for interaction with the environment. The term includes, without limitation, an irreversible vegetative state or irreversible coma.

person: Any individual, corporation, partnership, association, or other similar entity, or any federal, state, or local government or governmental agency.

principal: An individual who executes an advance health care directive, designates an individual to act or disqualifies an individual from acting as a health care representative, or an individual for whom a health care representative acts in accordance with this chapter.

reasonably available: Readily able to be contacted without undue effort and willing and able to act in a timely manner considering the urgency of the individual's health care needs.[24]

The requirements for writing a living will are that an individual must be of sound mind and be eighteen years of age or older (or be a high school graduate, be married, or be an emancipated minor). The living will must be dated and signed by the principal with either a signature or mark or by another individual on behalf of or at the direction of the principal if the principal is unable to sign. The living will must also be witnessed by two individuals, each of whom is eighteen years of age or older. It is also stipulated that an individual who signs a living will on behalf of the principal may not witness the living will. In addition, a health care provider (hospital, nursing home, or other) and its agents may not sign a living will on behalf of and at the direction of a principal if the health care provider or agent provides health care services to the principal. Once the living will is completed, the principal should give copies of it to those individuals who will be certain to present it to the attending physician or the health care provider when it is appropriate.[25] The principal should also sit down with these individuals and review the advance directive/living will with them to help eliminate any ambiguity about intention, wording, or wishes.

There are no specific guidelines for what the content of a living will should include. Bioethicist Mark Miller recommends three essential things that should be included in an advance directive/living will. "First, if you are dying (and unable to make your own decisions), ask for palliative or hospice care, which is treatment appropriate for the dying. Second, it is important to make a statement about your most fundamental beliefs. Third, it is helpful to put a 'safety valve' statement into one's advance directive/living will. 'If you do not know what my condition is, please treat me until you do know; then follow my wishes—make me better if you can, or allow me to die according to my instructions.'"[26]

Miller also believes there are certain specific issues that need to be considered concerning end-of-life choices: use of a ventilator, cardiopulmonary resuscitation (code status), surgery or aggressive medical interventions, and artificial hydration and nutrition.[27] All of these issues need to be considered, but it is important to state that one cannot cover every issue or condition that could arise. Making an advance directive/living will clear and specific to avoid ambiguity is good, but these documents are not foolproof.

For the living will to become operative, first, a copy of the document has to be given to the attending physician and placed on the principal's chart. Second, the attending physician must certify in writing that the principal is "incompetent" and has either an "end-stage medical condition" or is permanently unconscious. Finally, once it is determined that the living will is operative, the attending physician and other health care providers will act in accordance with its provisions. A surrogate, proxy, or durable power of attorney for health care cannot override an advance directive/living will if it has been declared operative.

If an attending physician or health care provider are unable in good conscience to comply with the provisions of the living will, that party is required to make every reasonable effort to assist in the transfer of the principal to another physician or health care provider who can comply with the living will. There are two exceptions to complying with an operative living will. The first is if 911 is activated and the principal does not have an out-of-hospital DNR order; the EMS personnel *will* give emergency treatment. Second, the law mandates the provision of life-sustaining medical treatment to an incompetent pregnant woman unless life-sustaining treatment will not maintain the pregnant woman in such a way as to permit the continuing development and live birth of the unborn child; or will be physically harmful to the woman; or will cause pain to the woman that cannot be alleviated by medication. These determinations must be made to a reasonable degree of medical certainty and certified by the woman's attending physician and an obstetrician who has examined the woman. Act 169 requires the state to pay for life-sustaining care provided to a pregnant woman under this provision.[28]

A patient may amend an advance directive or living will only if the patient is of sound mind. An amendment must conform to the requirements for executing an advance directive or living will. In the case of multiple advance directives or living wills, the latest directive prevails. An advance directive or living will may be revoked at any time and in any manner by the principal regardless of the mental and physical condition of the principal. Revocation of these documents is effective upon communication to the attending physician or other health care provider by the principal or a witness to the revocation. The attending physician or health care provider must make the revocation immediately part of the principal's medical record.[29] Many people in Pennsylvania question why the legislators allow for incompetent people to revoke their living will. The only possible explanation is that they are protecting the person's right of self-determination. This appears to be an extreme measure and not prudent under most circumstances.

Another major benefit of Act 169 is that it requires the Department of Health, in consultation with the advisory committee, to consider adoption of a standardized POLST (physician orders for life-sustaining treatment) form.[30] "The POLST form allows persons with serious medical conditions to document their advance decisions for life-prolonging treatments as clear, specific written medical orders, which will be honored in all settings."[31] This concept originated in Oregon and has spread to other areas including Western Pennsylvania. The first version of the form was implemented in 1995 (see Appendix H). "By 1998, early research confirmed that patients with POLST forms received the care they wanted and did not receive the care they did not want. In a study of 180 nursing home residents requesting comfort care measures only, transfer to hospital only if comfort measures fail, and do not resuscitate (DNR) orders, only 2 percent were hospitalized to extend their lives, and no one was resuscitated against patient's wishes.[32]

The reason the POLST form is so important is that it provides for the continuity of care, especially in regards to DNR orders and other life-sustaining treatment orders, from one setting to another. So, if a patient is transferred from a nursing home to a hospital, the POLST form is transferred with the patient to assure that each person's difficult decisions regarding end-of-life care are honored and are not dishonored due to misplaced or delayed paperwork. The Pennsylvania Medical Society is advocating for the POLST program in Pennsylvania.[33] The POLST form is currently being considered by an advisory committee of the Pennsylvania Department of Health.

Another type of advance directive/living will is a form called "Five Wishes." The Five Wishes document is unique among other living will forms because it looks at the total needs of the person: medical, personal, emotional, and spiritual. It allows you to choose the person you want to make medical decisions for you in the event that you become incompetent. It was designed and written with the help of the American Bar Association's Commission on the Legal Problems of the Elderly and the nation's leading experts in end-of-life care. Anyone eighteen years of age and older who is competent can write Five Wishes. The following five wishes let your surrogate, family members, and physicians know what you would want in the event that you become incompetent:

1. Which person you want to make health care decisions for you when you can't make them.
2. The kind of medical treatment you want or don't want.
3. How comfortable you want to be.
4. How you want people to treat you.
5. What you want your loved ones to know.

It is estimated that nearly six million copies of this document are circulating throughout the United States. Currently, a "Five Wishes" document meets the legal requirements under the health decisions statutes of thirty-six states and the District of Columbia.

Unfortunately, if you live in the state of Alabama, Indiana, Kansas, Kentucky, Nevada, New Hampshire, Ohio, Oklahoma, Oregon, South Carolina, Texas, Utah, Vermont, or Wisconsin, Five Wishes does not meet the technical requirements in the statutes of your state, and some doctors in your state may be reluctant to honor your Five Wishes. However, you can still use Five Wishes to put your wishes in writing. This will be a helpful guide to your surrogate, family members, and physicians. Most physicians and health care professionals understand that they have a duty to listen to your wishes no matter how you express them.[34]

Advance directives/living wills might make medical decision making at the end-of-life easier for loved ones. No matter how specific one might be in writing an advance directive/living will, these documents will always be ambiguous to a certain degree and can be misinterpreted. That is why these documents should be written in combination with the appointment of a durable power of attorney for health care. Appointing a person who knows the patient's values and wishes and will be able to carry out those wishes in the best interest of the patient can help to lighten the burden of end-of-life decision making for everyone involved.

DURABLE POWER OF ATTORNEY FOR HEALTH CARE

When a person is no longer competent, the patient's wishes are expressed by a substitute decision maker—that is, someone who knows the patient's wishes and values and makes medical decisions based on what he or she believes the patient would want if the patient were competent. Such a substitute decision maker is known by terms such as *durable power of attorney for health care*, *proxy*, *health care agent*, *patient surrogate*, and *next of kin*. Each of these terms refers to a person (or persons) who can make a substituted judgment for a patient who cannot make decisions, but the one with the most legal standing is the durable power of attorney for health care. A durable power of attorney for health care is a document that permits an individual, called a principal, to appoint or delegate another person (or persons) to make health care decisions for the principal in the event that the principal becomes incompetent.

In the state of Pennsylvania, any individual of sound mind and eighteen years of age or older (or who has graduated from high school, or is married, or is an emancipated minor) can appoint a durable power of attorney. The health care power of attorney (POA) form must be signed by the principal by a signature or a mark or by another person on behalf of and at the direction of the principal if the principal is unable to sign. It must also be witnessed by two individuals eighteen years of age or older (see Appendix I). As with the living will form, any individual who signs a health care power of attorney on behalf of or at the direction of a principal may not witness the health care power of attorney. A health care provider and its agents may not sign a health care power of attorney on behalf of or at the direction of a principal if the health care provider or its agents provide health care services to the principal.[35]

In choosing a health care POA, two things are essential. First, choose someone who knows your wishes and values. Second, choose someone you know is capable of carrying out your instructions if you should become incompetent. It is also imperative that you communicate to your physician and family the name of this person so that all parties know a decision maker is in place when a crisis arises.[36] The principal can give a health care POA authority as broad as the patient would have if competent. In contrast to living wills, health care POAs are not restricted to end-of-life decision making. Although they are usually given authority only when the patient is incompetent, a principal may invest a health care POA with authority even when the patient is competent. In the state of Pennsylvania, a health care POA cannot be the principal's attending physician, health care provider, or the owner, operator, or employee where a principal is receiving care unless related to the principal by blood, marriage, or adoption. Usually, the health care POA document only becomes operative when a copy is provided to the attending physician and the attending physician determines that the principal is incompetent. A copy of the health care POA document should be placed in the principal's medical record. [37]

The duty of a health care POA is to gather information about the principal's diagnosis, prognosis, and acceptable medical alternatives regarding diagnosis, treatments, and supportive care. The health care POA should make medical decisions in accordance with the POA's understanding and interpretation of the instructions given by the principal at a time when the principal had capacity to make and communicate such decisions. In the absence of such instructions, the health care POA should make medical decisions for the principal that conform with the principal's preferences and values, including religious and moral beliefs. If the principal's preferences are unknown, the health care POA should take into account what he or she knows of the principal's values and beliefs and assess what is in the principal's best interest and then decide, taking into consideration the following goals: the preservation of life; the relief of suffering; and the preservation and restoration of functioning, taking into account any concurrent disease, illness, or physical, mental, cognitive, or intellectual conditions that may have predated the principal's end-stage medical condition.

The health care POA is not prevented from consenting to health care administered in good faith pursuant to religious beliefs of the principal or from withholding consent to health care that is contrary to the religious beliefs of the principal. The health care POA has the same rights and limitations as the principal to request, examine, copy, and consent to the disclosure of medical or other health care information. A principal of sound mind may modify or revoke a durable power of attorney for health care in writing or by orally informing the attending physician or health care provider. The law also states that, regardless of the patient's mental or physical capacity, a principal may countermand the decision of a health care POA that would withhold or withdraw life-sustaining treatment, by personally informing the attending physician. If it is determined by a judge that a durable power of attorney is not acting in the best interest of the patient, said judge can remove the durable power of attorney and appoint a guardian ad litem for the patient.[38]

In the absence of a health care POA or if the POA is not reasonably available, the following classes, in descending order of priority who are reasonably available, may act as the patient's proxy in the state of Pennsylvania: 1) the spouse, unless an action for divorce is pending, and the adult children of the patient who are not the children of the spouse; 2) an adult child; 3) a parent; 4) an adult brother or sister; 5) an adult grandchild; 6) an adult who has knowledge of the patient's preferences and values, including but not limited to religious and moral beliefs. If none of these individuals can be reasonably located, then the patient's health care provider must seek a legal guardian from the courts.

The Pennsylvania law stipulates that if there is more than one member of a class who assumes authority and the members do not agree, the decision is made by the majority members of the class. If the members of the class are evenly divided, no decision shall be deemed acceptable until the parties resolve their disagreement. Notwithstanding such disagreement, nothing shall preclude the administration of health care treatment in accordance with the accepted standards of medical practice.[39] If the disagreement seems unable to be resolved, the health care provider can refer the situation to the courts to have a guardian appointed. In Pennsylvania, if the patient's living will is operative, a durable power of attorney for health care cannot countermand the wishes of a patient stipulated in a living will. (It should be noted that this may not be true for all states.)

If the attending physician or health care provider cannot in good conscience comply with the decision of the health care POA, the attending physician must inform the health care POA and then assist the health care POA in the transfer of the principal to another physician or health care provider who can comply with the wishes of the health care POA. If transfer is impossible, the provision of life-sustaining treatment to a principal will not subject an attending physician or health care provider to civil or criminal liability or administrative sanction. The Pennsylvania Health Care Act provides criminal and civil immunity for health care providers who: (1) participate in the withdrawal of life-sustaining treatment if the provider believes the wishes of the principal have been followed in good faith; (2) comply with the direction of someone who the health care provider believes has the authority to act for the principal so long as the direction is not clearly contrary to the advance directive or living will that has been delivered to the health care provider; (3) refuse to comply with the direction of an individual based on good faith belief that the individual lacks authority to act as the principal's health care agent or is not acting in accordance with the Health Care Act's provisions regarding the authority of health care agents or decisions by health care representatives; (4) refuse to comply with a direction or decision of an individual based on a good faith belief that compliance with the direction would be unethical or would result in medical care having no medical basis in addressing the medical need or condition of the individual provided that care; (5) comply with provisions of the Health Care Act regarding notification and transfer of a patient and with provisions related to certification of end-stage medical condition; or (6) comply with obligations to preserve life if the individual does not have an end-stage medical condition or is not permanently unconscious.[40]

It should be noted that Pennsylvania's new Health Care Agents and Representatives Act, besides recognizing health care POAs, also gives patients the flexibility to appoint a health care agent by any signed written document or by verbally telling the patient's health care provider or attending physician who the patient authorizes to make health care decisions on behalf of the patient should the patient become incompetent.[41] The state recognizes the importance of advance directives, living wills, and durable powers of attorney for health care, but it also recognizes that if an individual fails to have these documents, it is vital that an individual appoint a health care agent so that attending physicians, health care providers, and family members know, to the best of their ability, the wishes of the individual should that individual become incompetent. Pennsylvania legislators went out of their way to make this process as simple as possible for its citizens so that, in the event that a person becomes incompetent, all parties concerned will act in the best interest of the person.

In the end, there is no magic formula that will make perfect medical treatment decisions for someone who is incompetent and has an end-stage medical condition or is permanently unconscious. Rather, the goal is to do the best we can with the tools that have been given to us. DNR orders, advance directives/living wills, and durable powers of attorney for health care are all tools that direct physicians and family members to make medical decisions that are in a patient's best interest and comply with that patient's values and wishes.

Terminally ill patients and their family members and caregivers deserve a system better than the one currently available. "They depend on the health care system to serve their needs and certainly not to add to the burden of their or a loved one's final days."[42] Meeting the needs of patients and family members will require initiating conversations about end-of-life treatment and care, understanding and respecting the values and wishes of the patient, confronting the barriers to respecting the patient's values and wishes, and developing new tools and policies to change the present health care system. Addressing these challenges will not only allow the terminally ill patient to die with dignity and respect, but will also give family members the peace of mind of knowing that they made decisions in the best interest of their loved one.

Do Not Resuscitate (DNR) Order

I, _____, (print full name) DO NOT
AUTHORIZE CARDIOPULMONARY RESUSCITATION.
I (or my legal representative) understand that this order remains in effect until revoked by me (or my legal representative) or the attending physician. I (or my legal
representative) acknowledge that cardiopulmonary resuscitation (CPR) will not
be performed if breathing or heart beat stops. (The signatures of [a] the patient OR
legal representative, [b] the physician and [c] two witnesses are required.)

_____ _____ _____
Printed name of patient   Signature of patient   Date

_____ _____ _____
Printed name of physician Signature of physician   Date

_____
Effective date

Legal Representative's Signature of Consent for Patient Lacking Decision-Making
Capacity (If the patient lacks decision-making capacity, then a signature in this
section is required.)

_____
Printed name of (circle appropriate title) legal guardian
OR durable power of attorney for health care agent
OR surrogate decision maker

_____
Street Address

_____

City, State, ZIP

_____

Signature of legal representative

_____

Date

_____   _____   _____

Printed name of witness   Signature of witness   Date

_____

Address of witness

_____   _____   _____

Printed name of witness   Signature of witness   Date

_____

Address of witness

Illinois Department of Public Health
535 W. Jefferson St.
Springfield, IL 62761
217-785-2080,
TTY (hearing impaired use only)
800-547-0466
Reproduce on brightly colored orange paper

Appendix B:
Sample DNR Order Sheet

DO-NOT-RESUSCITATE ORDER

I request that in the event my heart and breathing should stop, no person shall attempt to resuscitate me. This order is effective until it is revoked by me.

Being of sound mind, I voluntarily execute this order, and I understand its full import.

_____   _____
(Declarant's signature and Date)

_____
(Type or print declarant's full name)

_____   _____
(Signature of person who signed for declarant, if applicable, and Date)

_____
(Type or print full name)

ATTESTATION OF WITNESSES

The individual who has executed this order appears to be of sound mind, and under no duress, fraud, or undue influence. Upon executing this order, the individual has (has not) received an identification bracelet.

_____   _____
(Witness signature)   (Date)

93

_____

(Type or print witness's name)

_____

(Witness signature) (Date)

_____

(Type or print witness's name)

THIS FORM WAS PREPARED PERSUANT TO, AND IN COMPLI-
ANCE WITH, THE MICHIGAN DO-NOT-RESUSCITATE PROCE-
DURE ACT.

APPENDIX C:
SAMPLE DNR ORDER SHEET
THAT ALLOWS FOR A LIMITED CODE STATUS

PHYSICIAN ORDERS SHEET

CARDIOPULMONARY RESUSCITATION ORDER SHEET

____ No Cardiopulmonary Resuscitation/continue comfort measures

____ Limited Cardiopulmonary Treatment (specify)

_____

____ withhold antiarrhythmic drugs

____ withhold cardioversion/defibrillation/external pacing

____ withhold chest compressions

____ withhold intravenous vasopressor drugs

____ withhold endotracheal intubation

____ withhold mechanical ventilation

Procedures:

Discussed treatment and potential choices with patient and/or family/ guardian

95

Discussed with_____

Documented discussion in progress notes

Date _____

Signature of Attending Physician/Designee

_____

APPENDIX D:
SAMPLE AND/DNR ORDER SHEET

CARDIOPULMONARY RESUSCITATION ORDER SHEET

Code Status:

[ ]   AND—Allow Natural Death / DNR (Do Not Resuscitate)/ Continue Comfort Measures, No Cardiopulmonary Resuscitation/No Intubation or Mechanical Ventilation

[ ]   Perform Basic Cardiopulmonary Resuscitation/Withhold Endotracheal Intubation/Mechanical Ventilation

[ ]   Full Cardiopulmonary Resuscitation

Discussion/Content:

[ ]   Discussed treatment and potential choices with patient and/or authorized representative of the patient

[ ]   Documented discussion in Progress Notes Date:_____

Signature of Attending Physician/Designee:

_____Date:_____

_____Date:_____

N.B. Re-evaluate prior to and after going to the OR or Cathlab.

97

APPENDIX E:
SAMPLE EMERGENCY MEDICAL
PREHOSPITAL DNR FORM

**EMERGENCY MEDICAL SERVICES PREHOSPITAL DO NOT
RESUSCITATE (DNR) FORM**

An Advance Request to Limit the Scope of Emergency Medical Care

I, _____, request limited emergency
  (Print patient's name and medical record number)   care as herein described.

I understand DNR means that, if my heart stops beating or if I stop breathing, no medical procedure to restart breathing or heart functioning will be instituted.

I understand this decision will not prevent me from obtaining other emergency medical care by pre-hospital emergency medical care personnel and/or medical care directed by a physician prior to my death.

I understand I may revoke this directive at any time by destroying this form and removing any "DNR" medallions.

I give permission for this information to be given to the prehospital emergency care personnel, doctors, nurses, or other health personnel as necessary to implement this directive.

I hereby agree to the "Do Not Resuscitate" (DNR) order.

_____   _____

Patient/Surrogate Signature   Date

_____   _____

Print Surrogate's name   Relationship to Patient   Surrogate's phone number

By signing this form, the surrogate acknowledges that this request to forego resuscitative measures is consistent with the known desires of and with the best interest of the individual who is the subject of this form.
I affirm that this patient/surrogate is making an informed decision and that this di-

99

rective is the expressed wish of the patient/surrogate. A copy of this form is in the patient's permanent medical record.

In the event of cardiac or respiratory arrest, no chest compressions, assisted ventilations, intubation, defibrillation, or cardiotonic medications are to be initiated.

_____   _____
Physician Signature   Date

_____   _____
Print Name   California License number

THIS FORM WILL NOT BE ACCEPTED IF IT HAS BEEN AMENDED OR ALTERED IN ANY WAY

PREHOSPITAL DNR REQUEST FORM

Original is to be kept by patient. Submit a copy to be kept in patient's permanent medical record. If an authorized DNR medallion is desired, submit a copy of this form, with Medic Alert enrollment form, to Medic Alert Foundation, 2323 Colorado Avenue, Turlock, CA 95381. To obtain the Medic Alert enrollment form, call 1-800-432-5378.

APPENDIX F:
SAMPLE PENNSYLVANIA OUT-OF-HOSPITAL DO-NOT-RESUSCITATE ORDER

OUT-OF-HOSPITAL
DO-NOT-RESUSCITATE ORDER

PATIENT'S NAME:

_____

2A. Attending Physician Statement:

I, the undersigned, state that I am the attending physician of the patient named above. The above-named patient, or the patient's surrogate or other person by virtue of that person's legal relationship to the patient, has requested this order, and I have made a determination that this patient is eligible for an order and satisfies one of the following: (1) the patient has an end-stage medical condition; (2) the patient is in a terminal condition; (3) the patient is permanently unconscious and has a living will directing that no cardiopulmonary resuscitation be provided to the patient in the event of the patient's cardiac or respiratory arrest; or (4) the patient is permanently unconscious and has a living will authorizing the surrogate or other person named below to request an out-of-hospital do-not-resuscitate order for the patient. I direct any and all emergency medical services personnel, commencing on the date of my signature below, to withhold cardiopulmonary resuscitation, (cardiac compression, invasive airway techniques, artificial ventilation, defibrillation and other related procedures) from the patient in the event of the patient's respiratory or cardiac arrest. If the patient is not yet in cardiac or respiratory arrest, I further direct such personnel to provide to the patient other medical interventions, such as intravenous fluids, oxygen or other therapies necessary to provide comfort, care or to alleviate pain, unless directed otherwise by the patient or the emergency medical services provider's authorized medical command physician.

_____Printed:_____
Signature of Physician
Date: _____

Emergency Telephone Number:_____

Bracelet issued: _____Yes _____No   Necklace issued: _____Yes _____No

2B. Attending Physician Statement for Patient Pregnant When Order Issues (in addition to above statement):

I, the undersigned, certify that an obstetrician has examined the patient named above and that the obstetrician and I have certified in the patient's medical record as required by law that life-sustaining treatment, nutrition, hydration, and cardiopulmonary resuscitation will have one of the following consequences if provided to this pregnant patient: (1) they will not maintain the pregnant patient in such a way as to permit the continuing development and live birth of the unborn child; or (2) they will be physically harmful to the pregnant patient; or (3) they will cause pain to the pregnant patient which cannot be alleviated by medication.

Signature of Physician:

_____Printed:_____

Date: _____

3A. Patient's or Surrogate's Statement:

I, the undersigned, hereby direct that in the event of my cardiac and/or respiratory arrest efforts at cardiopulmonary resuscitation not be initiated and that they may be withdrawn if initiated. I understand that I may revoke these directions at any time by giving verbal instructions to the emergency medical services providers, by physical cancellation or destruction of this form or my bracelet or necklace or by simply not displaying this form or the bracelet or the necklace for my EMS caregivers.

Date_____   _____

                          Signature of Patient   (If patient qualified to sign)

3B. Surrogate's/other Person's (by virtue of relationship to patient) Statement:

I, the undersigned, hereby certify that I am legally authorized to execute this order on the patient's behalf by virtue of having been designated as the patient's surrogate and/or by virtue of my relationship to the patient (specify relationship: _____). I hereby direct that in the event of the patient's cardiac and/or respiratory arrest, efforts at cardiopulmonary resuscitation not be initiated and be withdrawn if initiated.

Signature of Surrogate/Other Person   Date
by Virtue of Relationship to Patient
(if patient not qualified to sign)

Out-Of-Hospital Do-Not-Resuscitate Order Information

Authority: Out-of-Hospital No Resuscitation Act (Act), P.L. 1484, No. 169 (20 Pa.C.S. §§ 5481-5488), effective January 28, 2007.

When Order is Effective: An out-of-hospital do-not-resuscitate (DNR) order is effective when it is signed by the attending physician. The attending physician signs last. It remains in effect until the death of the patient or the order is revoked.

Implementation: Emergency medical services (EMS**)** providers are obligated to honor an out-of-hospital DNR order when displayed with the patient or the patient is wearing an out-of-hospital DNR bracelet or necklace. Patient interventions indicated and not indicated under out-of-hospital DNR order:

Shall not be provided if patient is in cardiac or respiratory arrest:
CPR
Endo-tracheal intubation
Bag valve mask
Defibrillation
Common medications used during resuscitation efforts

Shall be provided if patient is not yet in cardiac or respiratory arrest*:
Oxygen
Suctioning
Medications and other interventions within scope of practice and as authorized by protocols or medical command orders, to provide comfort, care or alleviate pain
*These interventions are not to be provided if the patient or a medical command physician directs otherwise.

Pregnant patient: Statement 2B on the reverse side needs to be completed only if the patient is a woman and the physician diagnoses the woman to be pregnant at the time the out-of-hospital DNR order is issued.

Revocation: The out-of-hospital DNR order may be revoked by destroying or not displaying the order, bracelet, and necklace, or by conveying the decision to revoke the order verbally or otherwise at the time the patient experiences cardiac or respiratory arrest. If the patient obtained the out-of-hospital DNR order, only the patient may revoke it. If a surrogate/other person by virtue of relationship to the patient obtained the out-of-hospital DNR order, the patient or a surrogate/other person by virtue of relationship to patient may revoke the order. Neither the patient's mental or physical condition limits the patient's right to revoke an out-of-hospital DNR order.

Definitions:

Out-of-hospital DNR patient: A patient for whom an attending physician has issued an out-of-hospital DNR order.

Surrogate: A "health care agent" or a "health care representative" as those terms are defined in 20 Pa.C.S. § 5422.

Attending physician: A physician who has primary responsibility for the medical care and treatment of a patient. A patient may have more than one attending physician.

End-stage medical condition: An incurable and irreversible medical condition in an advanced state caused by injury, disease, or physical illness which will, in the opinion of the attending physician, to a reasonable degree of medical certainty, result in death despite the introduction or continuation of medical treatment.

EMS provider: An ambulance attendant, first responder, EMT, paramedic, pre-hospital registered nurse, health professional physician, medical command physician, advanced life support service medical director, medical command facility medical director, medical command facility, ambulance service and quick response service as defined in regulations adopted under the Emergency Medical Services Act, and an individual who is given good Samaritan civil immunity under 42 Pa.C.S. § 8331.2 (when using an automated external defibrillator).

Out-of-hospital DNR order: A written order that is issued by an attending physician and directs EMS providers to withhold or withdraw CPR from the patient in the event of cardiac or respiratory arrest. The form for the physician's order is supplied by the Department of Health or its designee.

Permanently unconscious: A medical condition that has been diagnosed in accordance with currently accepted medical standards and with reasonable medical certainty as total and irreversible loss of consciousness and capacity for interaction with the environment. The term includes, without limitation, an irreversible vegetative state or irreversible coma.

Terminal condition: An incurable and irreversible medical condition in an advanced state caused by injury, disease or physical illness which will, in the opinion of the attending physician, to a reasonable degree of medical certainty, result in death regardless of the continued application of life-sustaining treatment.

HEALTH CARE TREATMENT INSTRUCTIONS IN THE EVENTOF END-STAGE MEDICAL CONDITION OR PERMANENT UNCONSCIOUSNESS (LIVING WILL)

The following health care treatment instructions exercise my right to make my own health care decisions. These instructions are intended to provide clear and convincing evidence of my wishes to be followed when I lack the capacity to understand, make, or communicate my treatment decisions:

IF I HAVE AN END-STAGE MEDICAL CONDITION (WHICH WILL RESULT IN MY DEATH, DESPITE THE INTRODUCTION OR CONTINUATION OF MEDICAL TREATMENT) OR AM PERMANENTLY UNCONSCIOUS SUCH AS AN IRREVERSIBLE COMA OR AN IRREVERSIBLE VEGETATIVE STATE AND THERE IS NO REALISTIC HOPE OF SIGNIFICANT RECOVERY, ALL OF THE FOLLOWING APPLY **(CROSS OUT ANY TREATMENT INSTRUCTIONS WITH WHICH YOU DO NOT AGREE):**

1. I direct that I be given health care treatment to relieve pain or provide comfort even if such treatment might shorten my life, suppress my appetite or my breathing, or be habit-forming.
2. I direct that all life-prolonging procedures be withheld or withdrawn.
3. I specifically do not want any of the following as life-prolonging procedures: (If you wish to receive any of these treatments, write **"I do want"** after the treatment)

        heart-lung resuscitation (CPR)_____

        mechanical ventilator (breathing machine)_____

        dialysis (kidney machine)_____

        surgery _____

        chemotherapy _____

        radiation treatment_____

        antibiotics_____

        Please indicate whether you want nutrition (food) or hydration (water)

medically supplied by a tube into your nose, stomach, intestine, arteries, or veins if you have an end-stage medical condition or are permanently unconscious and there is no realistic hope of significant recovery.
(Initial only one statement.)

TUBE FEEDINGS
_____I want tube feedings to be given

OR

NO TUBE FEEDINGS
_____I do not want tube feedings to be given.

HEALTH CARE AGENT'S USE OF INSTRUCTIONS
(INITIAL ONE OPTION ONLY.)

_____My health care agent must follow these instructions.

OR

_____These instructions are only guidance. My health care agent shall have final say and may override any of my instructions. (Indicate any exceptions.)

_____

–

_____

–

_____

–

If I did not appoint a health care agent, these instructions shall be followed.

LEGAL PROTECTION

Pennsylvania law protects my health care agent and health care providers from any legal liability for their good faith actions in following my wishes as expressed in this form or in complying with my health care agent's direction. On behalf of myself, my executors and heirs, I further hold my health care agent and my health care providers harmless and indemnify them against any claim for their good faith actions in recognizing my health care agent's authority or in following my treatment instructions.

ORGAN DONATION (INITIAL ONE OPTION ONLY.)

_____I consent to donate my organs and tissues at the time of my death for the purpose of transplant, medical study, or education. (Insert any limitations you desire on donation of specific organs or tissues or uses for donation of organs and tissues.)

_____

_____

_____

OR

_____I do not consent to donate my organs or tissues at the time of my death.

Having carefully read this document, I have signed it this ____ day of _____, 20___, revoking all previous health care powers of attorney and medical health care treatment instructions.

_____

Signature

WITNESS: _____
Address of Witness:

_____

WITNESS: _____
Address of Witness:

_____

Two witnesses at least 18 years of age are required by Pennsylvania law and should witness your signature in each other's presence. A person who signs this document on behalf of and at the direction of a principal may not be a witness. (It is preferable if the witnesses are not your heirs, nor your creditors, nor employed by any of your health care providers.)

NOTARIZATION (OPTIONAL)
 (Notarization of document is not required by Pennsylvania law, but if the document is both witnessed and notarized, it is more likely to be honored by the laws of some other states.)

On this____ day of_____ , 20____, before me personally appeared the aforesaid declarant and principal, to me known to be the person described in and who executed the foregoing instrument and acknowledged that he/she executed the same as his/her free act and deed.

IN WITNESS WHEREOF, I have hereunto set my hand and affixed my official seal in the
County of_____, State of _____ the day and year first above written.

_____   _____
Notary Public   My commission expires

APPENDIX H:
SAMPLE POLST FORM

Physician Orders for Life-Sustaining Treatment	Last Name
(POLST) First follow these orders, then contact physician or NP.	First Name/Middle Initial
This is a Physician Order Sheet based on the person's medical condition and wishes. Any section not completed implies full treatment for that section. Everyone shall be treated with dignity and respect.	Date of Birth

A

Check One

CARDIOPULMONARY RESUSCITATION (CPR): Person has no pulse and is not breathing. Resuscitate/CPR Do Not Attempt Resuscitation (DNR/no CPR) When not in cardiopulmonary arrest, follow orders in **B**, **C** and **D**.

B

Check One

© **CENTER FOR ETHICS IN HEALTH CARE, OHSU** Form developed in conformance with Oregon Revised Statute 127.505 et seq September 2004

C

Check One

ANTIBIOTICS No antibiotics. Use other measures to relieve symptoms. Determine use or limitation of antibiotics when infection occurs. Use antibiotics if life can be prolonged. Additional Orders:

D

Check One

Additional Orders: No artificial nutrition by tube. Defined trial period of artificial nutrition by tube. Long-term artificial nutrition by tube. **ARTIFICIALLY ADMINISTERED NUTRITION: Always offer food by mouth if feasible.**

E   SUMMARY OF MEDICAL CONDITION AND SIGNATURES

Discussed with: Patient Parent of Minor
Health Care Representative Court-Appointed
Guardian Other:
Summary of Medical Condition
Print Physician/ Nurse Practitioner Name
MD/DO/NP Phone Number
Office Use Only

Physician/ NP Signature (mandatory)	Date

SEND FORM WITH PERSON WHENEVER TRANSFERRED OR DISCHARGED

© **CENTER FOR ETHICS IN HEALTH CARE,** Oregon Health & Science University, 3181 Sam Jackson Park Rd, UHN-86, Portland, OR 97239-3098 (503) 494-3965
This POLST form is provided as a sample only and is not to be reproduced for patient use.
HIPAA PERMITS DISCLOSURE OF POLST TO OTHER HEALTH CARE PROFESSIONALS AS NECESSARY

Signature of Person, Parent of Minor, or Guardian/Health Care Representative

Significant thought has been given to life-sustaining treatment. Preferences have been expressed to a physician and/or health care professional(s). This document reflects those treatment preferences. (If signed by surrogate, preferences expressed must reflect patient's wishes as best understood by surrogate.)

Signature (optional)	Name (print)	Relationship (write "self" if patient)

Contact Information

Surrogate (optional)	Relationship	Phone Number	
Health Care Professional Preparing Form (optional)	Preparer Title	Phone Number	Date Prepared

Directions for Health Care Professionals Completing POLST Must be completed by a health care professional based on patient preferences and medical indications. POLST must be signed by a physician or nurse practitioner to be valid. Verbal orders are acceptable with follow-up signature by physician or nurse practitioner in accordance with facility/community policy. Use of original form is strongly encouraged. Photocopies and FAXes of signed POLST forms are legal and valid. **Using POLST** Any incomplete section of POLST implies full treatment for that section. No defibrillator (including AEDs) should be used on a person who has chosen "Do Not Attempt Resuscitation." Oral fluids and nutrition must always be offered if medically feasible. When comfort cannot be achieved in the current setting, the person, including someone with "Comfort Measures Only," should be transferred to a setting able to provide comfort (e.g., treatment of a hip fracture). IV medication to enhance comfort may be appropriate for a person who has chosen "Comfort Measures Only." Treatment of dehydration is a measure which prolongs life. A person who desires IV fluids should indicate "Limited Interventions" or "Full Treatment." A person with capacity, or the surrogate of a person without capacity, can request alternative treatment. **Reviewing POLST** This POLST should be reviewed periodically and if: (1) The person is transferred from one care setting or care level to another, or (2) There is a substantial change in the person's health status, or (3) The person's treatment preferences change. Draw line through sections A through E and write "VOID" in large letters if POLST is replaced or becomes invalid.

The POLST program was developed by the Oregon POLST Task Force. The POLST program is administratively housed at Oregon Health & Science University's Center for Ethics in Health Care. Research about the safety and effectiveness of the POLST program is available online at <**www.polst.org**> or by contacting the Task Force at <**polst@ohsu.edu**>. **The Oregon POLST Task Force.**
SEND FORM WITH PERSON WHENEVER TRANSFERRED OR DISCHARGED

MEDICAL INTERVENTIONS: Person has pulse and/or is breathing. Comfort Measures Only Use medication by any route, positioning, wound care and other measures to relieve pain and suffering. Use oxygen, suction and manual treatment of airway obstruction as needed for comfort. **Do not transfer** to hospital for life-sustaining treatment. **Transfer** if comfort needs cannot be met in current location. **Limited Additional Interventions** Includes care described above. Use medical treatment, IV fluids and cardiac monitor as indicated. Do not use intubation, advanced airway interventions, or mechanical ventilation. **Transfer** to hospital if indicated. Avoid intensive care. **Full Treatment** Includes care described above. Use intubation, advanced airway interventions, mechanical ventilation, and cardioversion as indicated. **Transfer** to hospital if indicated. Includes intensive care. Additional Orders:

Appendix I:

Sample Form, Durable Power of Attorney for Health Care

DURABLE POWER OF ATTORNEY FOR HEALTH CARE

I, _____, of _____ County, Pennsylvania, appoint the person named below to be my health care agent to make health and personal care decisions for me. Effective immediately and continuously until my death or revocation by a writing signed by me or someone authorized to make health care treatment decisions for me, I authorize all health care providers or other covered entities to disclose to my health care agent, upon my agent's request, any information, oral or written, regarding my physical or mental health, including, but not limited to, medical and hospital records and what is otherwise private, privileged, protected or personal health information, such as health information as defined and described in the Health Insurance Portability and Accountability Act of 1996 (Public Law 104-191, 110 Stat. 2024 1936), the regulations promulgated thereunder and any other State or local laws and rules. Information disclosed by a health care provider or other covered entity may be redisclosed and may no longer be subject to the privacy rules provided by 45 C.F.R. Pt. 164.The remainder of this document will take effect when and only when I lack the ability to understand, make, or communicate a choice regarding a health or personal care decision as verified by my attending physician. My health care agent may not delegate the authority to make decisions.

MY HEALTH CARE AGENT HAS ALL OF THE FOLLOWING POWERS SUBJECT TO THE HEALTH CARE TREATMENT INSTRUCTIONS THAT FOLLOW IN PART III (**CROSS OUT ANY POWERS YOU DO NOT WANT TO GIVE YOUR HEALTH CARE AGENT**):

1. To authorize, withhold, or withdraw medical care and surgical procedures.
2. To authorize, withhold, or withdraw nutrition (food) or hydration (water) medically supplied by tube through my nose, stomach, intestines, arteries, or veins.

3. To authorize my admission to or discharge from a medical, nursing, residential, or similar facility and to make agreements for my care and health insurance for my care, including hospice and/or palliative care.
4. To hire and fire medical, social service, and other support personnel responsible for my care.
5. To take any legal action necessary to do what I have directed.
6. To request that a physician responsible for my care issue a do-not-resuscitate (DNR) order, including an out-of-hospital DNR order, and sign any required documents and consents.

APPOINTMENT OF HEALTH CARE AGENT

I appoint the following health care agent:

HEALTH CARE AGENT:

_____
                    (Name and relationship)
Address: _____
Telephone Number: Home _____Work _____
E-MAIL: _____

IF YOU DO NOT NAME A HEALTH CARE AGENT, HEALTH CARE PROVIDERS WILL ASK YOUR FAMILY OR AN ADULT WHO KNOWS YOUR PREFERENCES AND VALUES FOR HELP IN DETERMINING YOUR WISHES FOR TREATMENT. NOTE THAT YOU MAY NOT APPOINT YOUR DOCTOR OR OTHER HEALTH CARE PROVIDER AS YOUR HEALTH CARE AGENT UNLESS RELATED TO YOU BY BLOOD, MARRIAGE, OR ADOPTION.

If my health care agent is not readily available or if my health care agent is my spouse and an action for divorce is filed by either of us after the date of this document, I appoint the person or persons named below in the order named. (It is helpful, but not required, to name alternative health care agents.)

FIRST ALTERNATIVE HEALTH CARE AGENT:

_____
                    (Name and relationship)
Address: _____
Telephone Number: Home_____ Work _____
E-MAIL: _____

SECOND ALTERNATIVE HEALTH CARE AGENT:

_____
(Name and relationship)
Address: _____
Telephone Number: Home_____ Work _____
E-MAIL: _____

FIVE:
PAIN MANAGEMENT

Humankind has been trying to understand pain since the beginning of human existence. "The philosophical, political, and religious meaning of pain defined the suffering of individuals for much of human history. Pain is the central metaphor of Judeo-Christian thought: the test of pain in the story of Job, the sacrificial redemption of the crucifixion. In the utilitarian dialectic of the eighteenth and nineteenth centuries, pleasure was balanced against pain to determine the good of society."[1] Pain has also been a medical problem. Physicians in Europe relieved pain in patients through the judicious use of opium, and after 1680 with the use of laudanum, a mixture of opium in sherry introduced by Thomas Sydenham.

Attitudes toward pain changed in the 1800s with the utilitarian emphasis on reducing pain for the greatest number of people and the new philosophy of individual rights. On October 16, 1846, William T. G. Morton, an American dentist, gave a demonstration of anesthesia with ether. And British obstetrician James Young proposed the use of chloroform in childbirth and surgery in 1848. The introduction of surgical anesthesia was a pivotal point in modern medicine, but this advancement did not come about without significant debate and controversy. The debates ranged from the ethics of operating on an unconscious patient to the possibility that the relief of pain might actually retard the healing process. Even some religious writers questioned whether anesthesia might be a violation of God's law, because they believed that God inflicted pain to strengthen faith and to teach a new mother the need for self-sacrifice for her children. Despite this controversy, surgeons used anesthesia to perform longer and more complex procedures, but for much of the nineteenth century it was not a universal practice. The gradual acceptance of surgical and obstetrical anesthesia promoted a general consensus that the relief of bodily pain was a positive good, if secondary to curative therapy.[2]

Pain became classified into three distinct categories: acute pain, severe pain in those suffering and dying from progressive diseases, and intractable chronic pain. Throughout the nineteenth century, opiates were the standard treatment for acute pain from injuries and for recurrent pain such as headache or toothache. Morphine was industrially produced in Germany in the 1820s and in the United States a decade later. In 1855, Alexander Wood devised a syringe with a hollow needle for subcutaneous injection, which was of immediate practical benefit. Opium and alcohol-based compounds in the form of liquids, pills, and "headache powders," were unregulated and available over the counter in local pharmacies. By the 1870s physicians began to express concerns about "the morphine habit" or "narcomania." In 1898, the Bayer Company of Germany introduced diacetylated morphine under the trade name of heroin as a cough remedy. It was less habit-forming than morphine. In 1899, Bayer introduced a new compound called aspirin, which proved to be remarkably safe and was well tolerated by patients. It was highly effective as an analgesic and antipyretic. For severe pain, however, opiates remained essential.[3]

Throughout the nineteenth century, physicians advocated the use of analgesics in seriously ill and dying patients. This was not universal, however, because of fears about the potential for addiction. The conflict between the physician's desire to relieve pain and fear of inducing addiction persisted in medicine throughout the twentieth century. There exists even today the fear of giving liberal amounts of narcotics which could lead to addiction. Some physicians even advised that every effort should be made to put off narcotic use until all other measures have been exhausted and the patient's life can be measured in weeks.[4]

"Research in the last thirty years has developed a variety of alternatives or adjuncts to opiates for chronic pain, including neuroactive medications, counterstimulation methods, and cognitive behavioral therapies."[5] The advancements in pain research and analgesic developments have not altered the truth of one clinical fact: "no one treatment works for every patient, even for pain of the same type and etiology. . . . The meanings of pain—cognitive, affective, behavioral—are different for each individual and shape the pain experience and response to therapy. . . . The most important treatment factor contributing to outcome was 'the intensive involvement of a single physician,' and why, with many new resources available, pain management remains a challenge for the clinician."[6]

The effective assessment and management of pain is a time-honored goal of medicine. From the time of Hippocrates[7] to the present-day *Code of Medical Ethics* of the American Medical Association,[8] the assessment and management of a patient's pain has been the primary responsibility of every physician. Nevertheless, due to various barriers, many patients today are not having their pain effectively assessed or managed. The 1995 SUPPORT study found that 50 percent of intensive care unit (ICU) patients suffered from moderate to severe pain during their last days of life. This study also found that pain assessment and management was not an institutional priority in most acute-care facilities.[9] Another report, by J. Lynn et al., shows that 40 percent of all dying patients in the United States die in pain.[10] In 1997, the Institute of Medicine found that anywhere from 40 to 80 percent of patients with terminal illness report that their treatment of pain is inadequate and prolongs the very agony of death.[11]

Older adults and those who are in a terminal condition are not alone in their struggle with pain. Schnitzer previously reported that 75 million American adults experience chronic pain.[12] "Dr. Russell K. Portenoy, chairman of pain medicine and palliative care at the Beth Israel Medical Center in New York, cites surveys estimating that as many as 6 to 10 percent of Americans suffer from chronic, disabling pain. He estimates that 1 in 10 of them could benefit from long-term, high-dose treatment."[13] Finally, a recent research study, directed by Dr. Joan Teno at Brown Medical School, on persistent pain in nursing home residents found that nationwide, 14.2 percent of residents, after two assessments, were in persistent pain, and 41.2 percent of residents in pain at first assessment were in severe pain 60 to 180 days later.[14] This high rate of persistent pain is consistent with other studies that have shown that pain is not adequately assessed or treated for patients in nursing homes.[15] The result of this undertreatment is impaired mobility, clinical depression, and a diminished quality of life for these patients.[16] These studies only confirm a long series of articles in the medical literature documenting the widespread and significant undertreatment of pain, beginning with a 1973 study of hospital inpatients.[17]

As a result of these studies, the Joint Commission on Accreditation of Health Care Organizations (JCAHO) was prompted to issue new revised standards, intent statements, scoring guidelines, and survey process questions so that they include assessment and treatment of pain in all patient populations.[18] The cornerstone of the revised JCAHO standards is that all patients have the right to appropriate assessment and management of pain and that this will be a condition of accreditation. Despite all this concern, the proper assessment and treatment of pain is still lacking in most of our acute-care facilities. Foley estimates that 60 to 90 percent of patients with advanced malignancy report significant pain.

Effective analgesic therapy is available, yet large segments of this population—in particular, elderly patients in nursing homes, minorities, and women—receive inadequate palliative care. In a recent Gallup poll, more than 70 percent of Americans surveyed said they still feared dying in pain and alone.[19] Even as recently as 2005, studies show that analgesic regimens are often inadequate, causing patients to experience unnecessary pain.[20] As a result, patients are pursuing other avenues to deal with the problem, such as litigation and the right to actively seek physician-assisted suicide.

Although the United States Supreme Court ruled in June 1997 that there was no federal or fundamental right to commit suicide, or thus, to have assistance in effecting it,[21] two concurring opinions by Justices O'-Connor and Stevens appear to legally validate the medical right to terminal sedation as an efficacious form of palliative treatment for intractable pain.[22] The Supreme Court put the medical profession on notice that it has a responsibility to relieve the pain and suffering of patients to the very best of their ability. If this cannot be done, then there is the distinct possibility that the discussion on physician-assisted suicide could be revisited by the Supreme Court. This warning, along with several recent court cases where family members successfully sued physicians for not adequately treating a patient's pain, demonstrate that in addition to representing an unacceptably poor quality of care, the undertreatment of pain may carry legal risks and consequences.[23]

These legal cases have placed the issue of pain assessment and management as a top priority in most acute-care facilities. But despite all this attention, there are still barriers that are causing patients not to have their pain adequately assessed and managed. This is not only a medical and legal issue, it is also an ethical issue. Patients have the ethical right to have their pain managed as part of the basic dignity and respect that is accorded to every human person. This right not only has a theological underpinning based in Scripture, especially the doctrine of Creation, it also has deep ethical roots in the medical profession. Some ethicists, such as Ben Rich, associate professor of bioethics at the University of California Davis Medical School, believe that the medical profession's failure to recognize the ethical implications of untreated and undertreated pain calls into question whether the majority of practitioners continue to acknowledge that health care is a moral enterprise.[24]

PROBLEMS RELATED TO PAIN ASSESSMENT AND MANAGEMENT

Pain is an unpleasant sensory and emotional experience.[25] It is recognized as a complex phenomenon derived from sensory stimuli and modified by individual memory, expectations, and emotions.[26] Since there are no objective biological markers of pain, the most accurate evidence of pain and its intensity is based on the patient's description and reporting. The dimensions of pain affect every person from the tiniest neonate to the elderly.[27] Pain can be classified into three categories, each of which can be acute or chronic. First, nociceptive pain is that generated by somatic or visceral tissue damage. Somatic pain is generated by nociceptors in cutaneous and deeper tissues (such as in the musculoskeletal system) and is described as gnawing, cramping, and throbbing. Visceral pain results from stimulation of the nociceptors in the cardiovascular, gastrointestinal, genitourinary, and respiratory systems. It is described as deep, aching, and squeezing, or as pressure. It is poorly localized and may be referred to cutaneous sites. Second, neuropathic pain usually is described as constant, burning, shooting, or lancinating (stabbing) pain. Third, incidental pain is pain secondary to associated conditions (not necessarily to cancer) such as positioning or constipation.[28]

Acute pain is pain that lasts or is anticipated to last a short period of time, typically less than one month. It is often associated with anxiety and with hyperactivity of the sympathetic nervous system. Chronic pain is usually defined broadly and arbitrarily as pain persisting for more than one month beyond the resolution of an acute tissue injury, pain persisting or recurring for more than three months, or pain associated with tissue injury that is expected to continue or progress. Chronic pain has no adaptive biologic role. Pain may be broadly classified as somatogenic (organic)—that is, explicable in terms of physiologic mechanism—or psychogenic, occurring without organic pathology sufficient to explain the degree of pain and disability and thought to be related mostly to psychological issues.[29]

Unrelieved pain is one of the greatest fears of people suffering from illnesses, especially terminal illness. Families of the suffering patient are in great distress, as well. This is in spite of the fact that 90 percent of the pain associated with severe illness can be relieved if physicians adhere to well-established guidelines and seek help, when necessary, from experts in pain management and palliative care.[30] Undertreatment of pain and unrelieved pain is also costly for patients, families, institutions, and society as a whole.[31] A 2003 study by Stewart et al. reported that between August

2001 and July 2002, an estimated 12.7 percent of the total U.S. workforce lost productive time over a two-week period because of pain, including headache (5.4 percent), back pain (3.2 percent), arthritis pain (2.0 percent), and other musculoskeletal conditions (2.0 percent). Of interest is that 80 percent of the lost productive time was explained by the reduced performance of work, not absence from work. In total, lost productive time cost employers an estimated $61.2 billion annually.[32] The reasons why pain has been undertreated or untreated are varied and numerous, but there are certain well-defined barriers that can be identified.

The barriers to effective pain assessment and management fall under four distinct categories. First, the failure of health care professionals to identify pain as a priority in patient care.[33] The failure of health care professionals to adequately treat pain is a result of a remnant of Cartesian dualism that dichotomizes the physical and the mental. Pain is the body's reaction to disease and suffering is the person's reaction to pain. Bodies are the site of disease, but persons undergo the experience of illness. Suffering is a personal matter. It is as much a function of the value of individuals as it is of its physical causes. Suffering is more global than pain and is synonymous with a reduced quality of life.[34] This dichotomy has allowed medical professionals to claim as their sole responsibility the treatment of the physical and biological domain of illness while surrendering the role of suffering to clinical psychologists, social workers, or pastoral counselors. The result of separating the objective dimension of disease from the subjective dimension of the person has been that the whole person's response to the experience of illness has been ignored, thus the failure of the medical profession to identify pain relief as a priority.[35]

Pain management should be a priority in the care of every patient and has deep roots in the medical profession. There have been notable advances in understanding pain in various stages of human development and significant improvements in pain management; the problem is that this knowledge has yet to affect routine clinical practices in many areas.[36i] Physicians have the responsibility to treat the patient and the person; that means they assess and manage every patient's pain and suffering, and if they fail to do so, they should be held accountable. Likewise, patients have a responsibility to make their physicians aware of the nature, severity, and duration of their pain to the best of their ability. The key is communication.

The best way to assess pain is to ask the patient. Since pain cannot be objectively quantified, physicians should believe their patients' accounts. Drug-seeking patients do exist, but they are a small minority. Patients need to be aware of the fact that they need not suffer; their pain can be and should be managed. This can be done on admission when the patient is informed, both orally and in writing, that effective pain relief is an important part of their treatment, that their communication of unrelieved pain is essential, and that health professionals will respond quickly to their reports of pain.[37] Unless there is open and honest dialogue between the patient and his or her physician, the covenant that binds them will be compromised through a breakdown of trust.

Second, there is insufficient knowledge among clinicians regarding the assessment and management of pain.[38] A major cause of this is the lack of education in medical schools regarding pain evaluation and management. A recent survey reported that the average amount of time spent teaching pain management in American medical schools was one hour, and for nursing schools it was four hours.[39] In addition, they receive one course in pharmacology, which cannot properly prepare them for what they will face once they leave the security of medical school. Once these individuals begin their residency and become attending physicians, it is almost impossible to keep abreast of the medical literature regarding pain management. There is a definite need for a comprehensive pain curriculum in every medical school.[40]

Critics of the medical school curriculum argue that when pain is addressed, too often it is by a faculty member whose knowledge and skills in assessment and management are woefully outdated, so that misinformation is passed from one generation of physicians to another virtually untouched by the remarkable advances of the last quarter century.[41] This becomes quite evident when doing rounds with medical interns and residents. They focus on the clinical problem, which might be a particular wound or the disease itself but fail to treat the entire patient.

Frequently, while doing ethics teaching rounds, a resident will present a case clinically and when he or she has finished, the bioethicist will ask, "What is being done for pain management with this patient?" Often, a blank stare accompanies the response: "I didn't think of that." Bioethicist Ben Rich believes this phenomenon might fairly be described as the "cultivation and propagation of ignorance."[42] If interns and residents have not been given the essential clinical competencies in pain management in medical school, and fail to receive these clinical competencies while in their residency programs, then when will they learn the importance of assessment and management of pain? One begins to wonder if pain management is a priority for physicians. One way to bring this issue to the forefront is the regular charting of a patient's pain as the "fifth vital sign." This could enhance the clinical competency of physicians in pain assessment and management and help to reassure patients that their fear of untreated pain will not become reality.

Third, there is a fear of regulatory scrutiny of prescribing practices for opioid analgesics.[43] Physicians are very open about the fact that they will underprescribe opioid analgesics to avoid regulatory scrutiny. Physicians fear not only government agencies such as the Drug Enforcement Administration (DEA) but also their own medical licensing boards. This fear among physicians is not only widespread; it is also based on factual evidence. "While the medical literature over the last quarter-century is replete with studies demonstrating widespread and significant underuse of opioid analgesics by physicians in their treatment of patients with pain, there is only a single instance in which a state board has disciplined a physician for unprofessional practice for failure to provide adequate pain management in the care of such patients. However, there are many cases in which the courts have criticized the efforts of state boards to discipline physicians on the grounds that they inappropriately prescribe (i.e., overprescribe) opioid analgesics for patients with pain."[44] It appears that the DEA has set the tone that drives physicians' perceptions about the legal risks associated with prescribing Schedule-II drugs (potentially addictive drugs with critical medical uses) for seriously ill and dying patients. Concerns about regulatory oversight have led some physicians to avoid prescribing opioids entirely and have rendered others fearful and hesitant.

Two recent attempts by the federal government to invalidate Oregon's "Death with Dignity Act" have only fueled this fear. In 1999, the "Pain Relief Promotion Act's" primary purpose was to make prescribing controlled substances under the Oregon law a violation of the "Controlled Substances Act." This act died in committee. Second, in November 2001, U.S. Attorney General John Ashcroft issued a directive suggesting that the prescription of Schedule-II medications under the Oregon law violates the "Controlled Substances Act" since assisting in a suicide is not a legitimate medical purpose. The U.S. Court of Appeals for the Ninth Circuit supported the arguments made by the State of Oregon and the case was appealed to the U.S. Supreme Court.[45] On January 17, 2006 the Supreme Court ruled in a six–three decision that the Oregon law trumped federal authority to regulate physicians.[46]

Despite the Supreme Court ruling, many physicians remain uncertain about prescribing opioids to control pain. Critics contend that the medical profession has been conscripted into the government's war on drugs. They contend that physicians believe their primary responsibility is to help regulators prevent drug diversion and excessive prescribing of opioid analgesics, not in effectively managing a patient's pain.[47] This fear, which is realistic, has resulted in physicians failing to act in the best interest of their patients. "A 1998 survey of more than 1,300 physicians by the New York State Medical Society found that 60 percent were moderately or very concerned about the possibility of being investigated by regulatory authorities for prescribing opiates for noncancer pain. A third said they prescribed lower qualities of pills at lower dosages 'frequently' because of the possibility of eliciting an investigation."[48]

As a result of this, the covenant between physician and patient can be fractured as the basic trust that held the covenant together dissolves. Both the state medical licensing boards and the federal government need to reevaluate and revise their present regulations regarding opioid analgesics. These antiquated regulations are causing patients to suffer needlessly, are raising the anxiety levels among those nearing death that the dying process will be cruel and full of excruciating pain, and are leading the American public toward the slippery slope of physician-assisted suicide. Instead of playing into this antiquated system of regulations, medical professionals should take the initiative to advocate for comprehensive new regulations.

There are also economic barriers to proper pain management. With the advent of managed care, there has been a greater inattention to pain assessment and management. Lower staffing levels, with fewer nurses having responsibility for a larger number of patients, decreases the likelihood that even a persistent patient will succeed in securing the required pain relief. The reluctance of physicians to prescribe and the lack of an adequate staff to monitor and evaluate patients will only lead to further barriers to pain relief for patients.[49]

Fourth, among health care professionals, there are persistent unsound beliefs and unsubstantiated fears about addiction, tolerance, dependence, and adverse side effects of opioid analgesics.[50] The major problem here is the lack of knowledge concerning the difference between addiction to narcotics and psychological dependence on opioid analgesics for relief of severe and persistent pain. The medical literature confirms that the majority of patients who receive large and extended doses of opioid analgesics for the management of their pain are not and rarely become addicts.[51] There is an abundance of medical literature emphasizing the important difference between the natural, physiological dependence that develops to opioid analgesics and the pathological, psychological dependence that characterizes addiction.[52]

"Physical dependence occurs in almost everyone who takes narcotic medication regularly for at least two weeks. Addiction is a craving for the drug and its compulsive use to regulate one's mood. With dependence, the body adapts physiologically to the drug, and if it is stopped abruptly, withdrawal symptoms occur. Tapering medications prevents nausea, vomiting, diarrhea, and cramping of withdrawal. Tolerance and physical dependence are normal and reflect the pharmacologic properties of opiates. People who are addicted to narcotics are generally dependent and tolerant, but dependence and tolerance only sometimes indicate addiction."[53]

It seems obvious that many physicians and nurses are not being exposed to this important medical information in their training. As a result, patients are being forced to endure unnecessary pain and suffering due to misinformation and ignorance. There are standard doses of commonly used opioids (see Appendix A). Guidelines have been established, and as long as a physician is acting in good faith and following the standard of care, addiction should not become an issue.

Another issue that physicians need to be more aware of and sensitive to is "breakthrough pain." Breakthrough pain is a flare of moderate to severe pain in patients with otherwise stable persistent pain. In other words, the intense pain "breaks through" the medication a patient is taking for persistent pain. Breakthrough pain typically comes on quickly, is very intense and lasts a relatively short period of time (up to an hour). Breakthrough pain often occurs without warning. Patients typically experience two to four episodes of breakthrough pain a day. Experts believe breakthrough pain is best treated with strong medications, such as an opioid, that acts quickly to relieve pain.

Researchers estimate that 64 percent of all cancer patients being treated for persistent pain experience breakthrough pain. Up to 74 percent of patients treated for pain stemming from other conditions (such as lower back pain, diabetic neuropathy, and osteoarthritis) experience breakthrough pain.[54] Medications for breakthrough pain, also known as "rescue medications," must be absorbed into the system rapidly to end short-term pain. It must also leave the patient's system quickly to avoid heightening side effects such as lethargy.

Traditional oral agents such as pills take fifteen to thirty minutes to reach peak levels and can also stay in the bloodstream for three to four hours. Medications administrated rectally (suppositories) work more quickly, but can be less desirable and less convenient. Research has shown that medication absorbed directly through the lining of the mouth (for example, rubbed along the inside of the cheek) is a good option for breakthrough pain relief. The only medication given this way is called oral transmucosal fentanyl citrate (OTFC, or the brand name: Actiq).

A new breakthrough pain medication for cancer patients is Fentora. It is a tablet placed between the upper cheek and the gum above the rear molar tooth. Fentanly, the pain-relieving ingredient in the tablet, is absorbed across the tissues, called the buccal mucosa, lining the upper cheek. According to the drug manufacturer, Cephalon, studies show that some patients experienced significant relief within fifteen minutes. Most short-acting opioids that are swallowed and absorbed through the stomach can take thirty to forty-five minutes to relieve pain.[55] Physicians and patients need to be aware that pain may arise when regular doses of medication for pain relief wear off. This in not considered breakthrough pain but may be a sign that the level of pain medication needs to be adjusted. Tolerance to pain medications is not uncommon in patients. Physicians need to be aware that breakthrough pain may be different for each person and is also often unpredictable. Breakthrough pain medications are necessary to control this type of pain and should be taken at the first sign of breakthrough pain.

Issues of patient tolerance to opioid analgesics are also based on myths and misinformation. The need for higher doses is almost invariably related to a progression of the underlying disease producing the pain. Patients whose disease is stable do not necessarily require an increase in dosage once an effective level of analgesic is achieved and maintained.[56] Finally, the issue of side effects from the sustained use of opioid analgesics has been greatly exaggerated according to pain management experts. The most common side effects of the drugs recommended for moderate to severe pain that persists are constipation, sedation, and respiratory depression. Prevailing clinical practice guidelines offer a range of effective means of managing these side effects without compromising the goal of pain relief.[57]

There are clear barriers to the assessment and management of pain that are complex and multifaceted, but they are not insurmountable. These barriers need to be challenged medically and ethically. If medicine is a moral enterprise, then there is not only a medical reason to challenge these barriers but also an ethical reason.

ETHICAL ANALYSIS

Failure to treat a patient's pain not only has medical implications but impacts on the deepest ethical roots of the medical profession. The primary responsibility of a physician is to do what is in the best interest of his or her patient. Not to treat the pain and suffering of a patient is to deny the patient's basic dignity as a human person. Failure of physicians to assess and adequately manage pain violates the basic ethical principles of respect for the human person, beneficence, nonmaleficence, and justice.

Respect for persons incorporates two ethical convictions: first, that individuals should be treated as autonomous agents; and second, that persons with diminished autonomy are entitled to protection. The principle of respect for persons thus divides into two separate moral requirements: the requirement to acknowledge autonomy and the requirement to protect those with diminished autonomy.[58] The physician–patient relationship is a covenant that is based on mutual trust. It is a fiduciary relationship based on honesty. Ethicists Edmund Pellegrino and David Thomasma, who have written extensively in this area, argue that among the obligations that arise from the physician–patient relationship is technical competence: "The act of the medical professional is inauthentic and a lie unless it fulfills the expectation of technical competence."[59] This means that patients can expect their physicians to have the technical skills to assess and manage their pain.

Unfortunately, most patients believe that the pain medications they are receiving are all the pain relief that can be safely and effectively administered. Therefore, they attribute their continued pain and suffering to the inherent limitations of medical science and technology.[60] This directly relates to the issue of informed consent. Patients have a right to be informed about the advantages and disadvantages of any treatment, as well as any viable alternatives. Patients cannot give informed consent, however, because in most cases they have not been given all the options available to manage their pain. Because of physicians' lack of education in pain management and the fear they have of regulatory scrutiny, patients are undertreated and their quality of life suffers.

One of the basic aspects of the principle of respect for persons is that a person should never be treated simply as a means, but always as an end. To undertreat a patient because of fear of regulatory scrutiny in prescribing opioid analgesics or out of misguided beliefs concerning addiction, dependence, and tolerance, is to treat that patient as a means rather than an end. Due to a basic lack of education, widespread misinformation, and unnecessary fear among physicians, patients are suffering needlessly, their autonomy is compromised, and the basic respect they deserve as human persons is violated—they are allowed to endure pain which can be alleviated. This violates the right of patients to be informed about their treatment options and to remain involved in the decision-making process.

Beneficence involves the obligation to prevent and remove harms and to promote the good of the person by minimizing possible harms and maximizing possible benefits. Beneficence includes *nonmaleficence*, which prohibits inflicting harm, injury, or death. In medical ethics, this principle has been closely associated with the maxim *Primum non nocere*—"Above all, do no harm." Allowing a person to endure pain when that pain can be managed and relieved violates the principle of beneficence because one is not preventing pain and therefore is not acting in the best interest of the patient. It also violates the principle of nonmaleficence because it is causing harm and even injury to the person. Prescribing lower doses of effective analgesics because the physician fears regulatory scrutiny, or failing to prescribe adequate doses of opioid analgesics because of misinformation about addiction, tolerance, and adverse side effects, places the patient in a situation in which his or her pain is either undertreated or not treated at all. This comes very close to willfully inflicting pain. It is true that most pain technologies also have risks of side effects associated with them. Therefore, the physician must balance the pain-relief potential with the potential harm. This can be done through dialogue with the patient and/or surrogates. The impact on the caregivers should also be considered in terms of physical and psychological burdens.[61]

Physicians have a moral obligation to do what is "good" for their patients. Compromising the basic ethical foundations upon which medicine stands is not only destructive for the patient but for society as a whole. It is true that patients have different pain levels that they can tolerate. It is also true that some people may wish to voluntarily embrace or tolerate suffering for spiritual reasons. For example, Christians believe that suffering can have value and is salvific, because the person experiences the love of Christ in a way that recalls Christ's own love as demonstrated in his willing acceptance of death on the cross. In this view, uniting one's suffering with Christ's is redemptive. This notion, however, should never be understood as a glorification of pain and suffering.

To endure *unnecessary* pain and suffering is not only useless, it is also a misrepresentation of the Christian position.[62] The Bishops of the United States in the *Ethical and Religious Directives for Catholic Health*

Care Services are quite clear that a patient's pain should always be managed effectively. "Patients should be kept as free of pain as possible so that they may die comfortably and with dignity, and in the place where they wish to die."[63] In fact, the Bishops go so far as to state that "medicines capable of alleviating or suppressing pain may be given to a dying person, even if this therapy may indirectly shorten the person's life, so long as the intent is not to hasten death."[64] This is justified under the principle of double effect.[65]

The use of morphine and the principle of double effect are two very important issues for patients and families in this area of pain management. Often, a patient or family member will express concern about the use of morphine because it could "kill" the patient. Morphine is an opium alkaloid and is the prototype of the opioid analgesics. In the nontolerant patient with severe pain, it provides pain relief at a dose of about 10 mg IM that does not result in severe alterations in consciousness. Morphine affects both the initial perception of pain and the emotional response to it. Total relief of pain is not always possible to achieve, but morphine can reduce the level of distress and suffering.

Traditionally, oral morphine has been considered to be ineffective. It is transformed rapidly in the liver and excreted in the urine. But with upward titration of the dose, oral morphine can be very effective in managing chronic pain. A slow-release tablet that dispenses morphine over eight to twelve hours and a concentrated oral solution have been developed in attempts to make oral morphine more acceptable. Morphine sulfate is the most commonly used water-soluble salt. Very low doses of intraspinal morphine (e.g., 5 to 10 mg epidurally, or 0.5 to 1 mg intrathecally) can provide long-lasting (up to 24-hour) pain relief postoperatively and in selected nontolerant cancer patients. To date, morphine is the drug most commonly used to manage pain for cancer patients.[66]

Adverse effects of morphine are related to dosage. These adverse effects include respiratory depression, decreased cough reflex, nausea, vomiting, constipation, itch, sedation, and confusion. Morphine can also produce miosis and can cause contraction of peripheral smooth muscle, the most important effect of which is decreased propulsive movements in the gastrointestinal tract, causing constipation. Morphine causes the venules (capacitance vessels) to dilate, and hypotension may occur in hypovolemic patients or in those who suddenly assume the upright position. The development of tolerance to morphine varies from one physiologic system to another (for example, tolerance develops slowly to the constipating effect, but respiratory depression or nausea typically wanes soon after treatment begins). During chronic therapy, an increase in dosage may become necessary to achieve the same degree of pain relief, since the duration of action shortens and the peak analgesic effect decreases.[67]

One major criticism of using morphine as a painkiller is that physicians often do not adequately explain to patients or their appropriate surrogate decision makers how morphine works and what its side effects can be. This is because many physicians are not adequately trained in the art of pain management. Instead of referring the terminal patient to a palliative care team which has expertise in pain management, the physician writes an order for morphine and the family is left to watch their loved one die. In many instances, patients and families are ill-prepared—emotionally and clinically—to make these decisions concerning the use of morphine. The result is that either the patient's pain is not managed adequately, or the families are left with feelings of guilt that they may have hastened their loved one's death. Family members may carry these feelings of guilt and frustration with them for a lifetime. Ethically, similar situations have led many health care professionals and other professionals to question the use of morphine as an effective way to manage pain in terminal patients.

The use of morphine is not only medically appropriate, it is also ethically and morally acceptable. The principle of double effect is a fundamental principle in Roman Catholic moral theology. As the name implies, it refers to one action with two effects. One effect is intended and is morally good; the other is unintended and is morally evil. It is not an inflexible rule or mathematical formula, but rather an efficient guide to prudent moral judgment in solving difficult moral dilemmas.[68] Historically, many ethicists believe the premises for the principle can be found in the writings of Thomas Aquinas in his famous explanation of the lawful killing of another in self-defense in the *Summa Theologicae* II, q. 64, a. 7c. Other ethicists argue that the four conditions of the principle were not finally formulated until the mid-nineteenth century by Jean Pierre Gury.[69] The principle of double effect specifies four conditions that must be fulfilled for an action with both a good and a bad effect to be morally justified.

1. The action, considered by itself and independently of its effects, must not be morally evil. The object of the action must be good or indifferent.
2. The evil effect must not be the means of producing the good effect.
3. The evil effect is sincerely not intended, but merely tolerated.
4. There must be a proportionate reason for performing the action, in spite of its evil consequence.[70]

It should be noted that a number of ethicists known as proportionalists have argued that the first three conditions of the principle of double effect are incidental to the principle, and that in reality it is reducible to the fourth condition of proportionate reason. While this is a legitimate argument, it is not the purpose of this chapter to reopen the controversy. This argument will remain within the framework of the four conditions of the principle of double effect, as it exists in fundamental moral theology, and will apply these conditions to the use of morphine as an ethical means of palliative care.[71]

The use of morphine to manage pain effectively is ethically justified because it meets the four conditions of the principle of double effect. The first condition allows for the injection of morphine because the action in and of itself is good, in that it effectively alleviates or manages the pain of the patient. While morphine may endanger the patient's life by suppressing respiration, the injection will not directly terminate the patient's life. The second condition allows for the injection of morphine because the good effect is not caused by means of the evil effect. The patient's pain is alleviated by the morphine not by the patient's death. The good effect and the evil effect happen simultaneously. The third condition allows for the injection of morphine because even though there is the possibility that the morphine may harm the patient, the intention of the physician is to alleviate or manage the patient's pain. Finally, the argument for the ethical justification of morphine for medical use by the principle of double effect focuses on whether there is a proportionately grave reason for allowing the foreseen but unintended possible consequences. Proportionate reason is the linchpin that holds this complex moral principle together.

Proportionate reason refers to a specific value and its relation to all elements (including premoral evils) in the action.[72] The specific value in using morphine and other pain analgesics is to relieve pain and suffering associated with treatment for specific illnesses. The premoral evil, which can come about by trying to achieve this value, is the foreseen but unintended possibility of the potential harmful effects of depressing the respiratory system and hastening death. The ethical question is this: Does the value of relieving pain and suffering outweigh the premoral evil of the potential harmful effects? To determine if a proper relationship exists between the specific value and the other elements of the act, ethicist Richard McCormick proposes three criteria for the establishment of proportionate reason:

1. The means used will not cause more harm than necessary to achieve the value.
2. No less harmful way exists to protect the value.
3. The means used to achieve the value will not undermine it.[73]

The application of McCormick's criteria to the use of morphine supports the argument that there is a proportionate reason for allowing physicians to prescribe it for palliative care. First, the use of morphine to control the pain and suffering in patients in certain situations does not cause more harm than necessary. With certain medical conditions, such as end-stage cancer, physicians will prescribe the use of morphine—even knowing the unintended side effects—because it is the only way to relieve the patient's pain. Not treating the pain and suffering of the patient would violate the right to being treated with dignity and respect. Second, when a patient is clearly in pain and all other medications do not relieve the pain, then the use of morphine is the only way to respect the value of the patient's life. Third, the use of morphine, if intended for palliative care, gives these patients the dignity and respect they deserve under these desperate conditions. Palliative care is given to respect the value of the patient's life. "Two million deaths a year occur in medical settings, and 85to 90 percent of those are preceded by decisions to withhold or end life support. The vast majority involve sedation."[74] Therefore, it would be ethically justified under the principle of double effect for medical professionals to give patients adequate doses of morphine or other pain medications if it is for palliative care. All individuals, but especially the seriously ill, have the right to effective pain management. To deny them access to such therapies is to deny them the dignity and respect all persons deserve. The greater good is promoted in spite of the potential evil consequences.

Another issue that has become prominent in recent years is that of "terminal sedation." It is also known as sedation of the imminently dying. Terminal sedation is a practice in which "(1) the patient is close to death (hours, days, or at most a few weeks); (2) the patient has one or more severe symptoms that are refractory to standard palliative care; (3) the patient's physician vigorously treats these symptoms with therapy known to be efficacious; (4) this therapy has a dose-dependent side effect of sedation that is a foreseen but unintended consequence of trying to relieve the patient's symptoms; and (5) this therapy may be coupled with the withholding or withdrawing of life-sustaining treatments that are ineffective or disproportionately burdensome."[75]

Terminal sedation is in direct contrast to "sedation toward death." This is a practice in which "(1) the patient need not be imminently dying; (2) the symptoms believed to be refractory to treatment are simply the consciousness that one is not yet dead; (3) the patient's physician selects therapy intended to render the patient unconscious as a means of treating the refractory symptoms; and (4) other life-sustaining treatments are withdrawn to hasten death."[76]

The principle of double effect applied to terminal sedation "maintains that it is not immoral to render a patient unconscious as a side effect of treating specific symptoms if (1) one does not aim at unconsciousness directly; (2) unconsciousness is not the means by which one intends to relieve symptoms; and (3) one has a 'proportionate reason' for taking such action. . . . The good effects must outweigh the bad and it must fit the situation."[77] This would not be the case for "sedation toward death" because the direct intention of the physician is to shorten the patient's life.

Physicians, as moral agents, have an ethical responsibility to treat their patients in a way that will maximize their benefits and minimize their harms. Failure to adequately assess and mange pain, for whatever reason, is not in the best interest of the patient. Therefore, if a physician has impediments to his or her reason or free will, due to fear or coercion, then that physician has an ethical responsibility to transfer his or her patient to a physician who will do what is demanded by the basic precepts of medicine—that which is for the good of the patient. This may mean having the courage to challenge state medical boards and the federal government to revise their regulations regarding opioid analgesics. Physicians who continue to remain uneducated about effective pain management, or who allow fear of regulatory scrutiny to guide their patient care, or who allow misinformation about opioid analgesics to continue to dominate their clinical practice have not only failed the test of beneficence, they have also failed the test of nonmaleficence.

Finally, the principle of *justice* recognizes that each person should be treated fairly and equitably, and should be given his or her due. Every patient has the right to have pain assessed and managed adequately. Some physicians are doing this well and others are failing. Whether this failure is because they lack the fundamental skills or essential clinical competencies, or because they fear government scrutiny of their methods, or simply because they are misinformed, it is inexcusable. Ignorance is not an excuse or a defense; physicians have the responsibility to be adequately trained and up-to-date on medications that will benefit their patients. If this is not possible, then these physicians have an ethical responsibility to consult those in the medical field who *are* trained to assess and manage pain effectively. To plead ignorance violates the very goals of medicine and the basic duty a physician has to his or her patients.

It has also been reported that two-thirds of pharmacies in minority neighborhoods do not carry adequate medications to treat persons in severe pain. This is a form of racial injustice according to Dr. Sean Morrison, a pain specialist at Mount Sinai School of Medicine in New York. Morrison and his colleagues surveyed New York pharmacies and found that, compared with white males, African Americans and Latinos do not get adequate treatment for severe pain. Not only are they less likely to be prescribed painkillers, but when they get a prescription, they may not be able to get it filled at a local pharmacy. In poor neighborhoods, pharmacists often decide not to stock opioids because of the risk of being targeted by drug addicts.[78] Pain is colorblind, and all people deserve to have their pain managed.

Health Care professionals have an ethical obligation to supply those medications needed to manage pain. To allow some patients, in similar situations, to be pain free and others to have their pain untreated or undertreated is an egregious violation of the principle of justice. Justice dictates that similar medical conditions should be treated in a similar manner if at all possible. If there are pain medications that can adequately manage pain for patients and these are prescribed for some, then failure to do so for all violates the basic tenet of justice, that is, to treat all fairly and equitably.

RECOMMENDATIONS:

The problems surrounding pain assessment and management are here to stay. Much has been written about the failure of health care professionals to address these issues, but simple rhetoric without significant reform will accomplish nothing. There is a need for immediate changes that will address the issues of pain assessment and management directly and concretely. If health care professionals honestly believe that one of the major goals of medicine is the relief of pain and suffering, then untreated and undertreated pain and unnecessary suffering have to be alleviated. Finally, if we know that our failure to relieve pain and suffering is causing people to seek other methods such as physician-assisted suicide, which we believe is unethical and immoral, then we must do everything in our power to help individuals deal with their pain and suffering in a way that benefits the good of the whole person. To accomplish this, I offer the following recommendations:

First, each hospital should formulate a pain management policy that will address the assessment and management of all types of pain. Appendix B, following this chapter, shows the pain management policy formulated by a Catholic health system. This policy is grounded in respect for the dignity of every human person and the duty of health care professionals to relieve the pain and suffering of patients.

Second, each hospital should also formulate a pain management team. This team should be interdisciplinary, consisting of a physician, nurse, social worker, physical therapist, pharmacist, anesthesiologist, psychiatrist/psychologist, pastoral care member, and someone skilled in alternative therapies. The purpose of this team is to assist physicians who are unable to manage a patient's pain. Any health care professional could request a pain consultation regarding a particular patient. The pain management team would inform the attending physician, evaluate the patient's situation, and then make specific recommendations on how to better manage the patient's pain. A pain management team is not only in the best interest of the patient, but also makes health care professionals more accountable for pain assessment and management.

Third, there is a need for more educational initiatives for health care professionals and the public regarding the way pain should be assessed and managed. This begins with medical schools instituting pain assessment and management curricula, residency programs that include practical experience in pain management (such as hospice), and the education of attending physicians through continuing medical education courses. This education of medical professionals must include instruction in pain assessment and management, pharmacologic principles, the uses of analgesics, and nonpharmacologic methods. There should also be education initiatives for the public.

The public should be educated to the fact that it can expect pain to be assessed and managed properly and that it too has a role to play in this process. Patients have the responsibility to report the nature, severity, and duration of their pain to their physicians and to expect that their pain will be relieved when possible. This can be accomplished by the regular charting of a patient's pain as the "fifth vital sign." It can also be accomplished by the staff instituting a simple assessment tool—a 0-to-10 pain-rating scale (or a "faces" scale for children and for those patients who are cognitively impaired).[79]

Fourth, physicians should begin a grass-roots movement to challenge the outdated regulations by medical boards and the federal government regarding opioid analgesics. If physicians are required to act in the best interest of their patients, then they should challenge—both as medical professionals and as ethical persons—the regulatory agencies that are hostile to effective pain management. Due to physician initiatives, "many legislatures and regulatory boards have adopted model pain statutes that encourage compliance with established standards for the prescribing of pharmacologic agents for pain and other symptoms and that protect physicians who observe these guidelines from regulatory intrusion and possible prosecution. Other states have simplified or eliminated special prescribing rules (such as those requiring the use of triplicate prescription pads) that were designed to control and monitor prescribing but that had the (presumably unintended) effect of discouraging all prescribing of controlled substances. California now requires training in pain management and palliative care as a condition of licensure."[80]

In 1998 the Federation of State Medical Boards, which represents American licensing boards, published "Model Guidelines for the Use of Controlled Substances for the Treatment of Pain" to assure physicians that appropriate prescribing of opioid painkillers would not lead to action against their licenses. Kansas was among the first states to adopt the guidelines. Now, twenty-two out of seventy American medical licensing authorities have done so. California also recently passed a bill called "The Medical Crimes: Investigations and Prosecutions." It requires that the state's district attorneys' association collaborate with "interested parties" on protocols to investigate physicians. Other states should follow suit and go even further by requiring prosecutors first to obtain declarations from qualified medical experts as to the good faith of the physician in question before charges are filed. It would go a long way toward making pain medication what it should be: a health care story, not a crime story.[81]

Pain is subjective and physicians have to rely on what their patients tell them. The DEA and other regulatory boards need to be aware of this fact and have to realize how tricky these medical judgments can be regarding pain medications. In general, regulatory oversight for prescribing opioids and other controlled substances should be viewed as educational and instructive not as punitive and disciplinary.

Fifth, more research and testing needs to be done to augment the pain medications available today for patients experiencing various types of pain. Researchers are trying to more precisely identify targets for pain therapy. The goal is to understand pain at a molecular level so that they can develop treatments aimed at specific molecules in pain pathways that relieve pain without causing adverse effects. Investigators are deciphering the ways pain travels from the periphery to the brain and back. They are identifying hundreds of players, including receptors that either facilitate or block pain perception, ligands (the molecules that bind to receptors or other targets), and other molecules that transmit signals to different cells. Research is also illuminating previously unsuspected roles played by nonneuronal cells and is uncovering genes that contribute to individual differences in the perception of pain.[82]

Researchers are also looking more carefully at the connection between physical and emotional pain. For decades, physicians have known that physical pain and depression are intertwined. Chronic pain can cause depression, while depression can heighten pain. In fact, up to 80 percent of patients with depression present with mainly physical symptoms. More research needs to be done in this area. Research into the connection between depression and the so-called monoamine neurotransmitters, serotonin and norepinephrine, should be pursued as well.[83] More research in these areas and especially at the molecular level means targeting specific mechanisms of pain rather than designing treatments for specific pain syndromes such as arthritis or diabetic neuropathy.[84] This will be far more advantageous to patients.

The issue of pain assessment and management is now a priority as it should always have been in the medical profession. Efforts must continue in order to advance knowledge about the mechanisms of pain, develop new and better analgesic medications and methods of delivery, remove the obstacles that prevent physicians from using known effective means of relieving pain in the very young, and educate patients and surrogates about effective use of pain-relieving therapies.[85] Reforms are needed from various aspects of society. It is both the professional and ethical responsibility of health care professionals to see that these reforms are initiated and carried out so that the best interest of the patient remains at the forefront of the medical profession. Pain management can be improved if it becomes a priority for all.

APPENDIX A:
STANDARD DOSES OF COMMONLY USED OPIOIDS*

Generic Name (Trade Name)	Analgesic Dose	Typical First Dose
Codeine		
Oral	30 mg every 3–4 hr	30 mg every 3–4 hr
Parenteral	10 mg every 3–4 hr	10 mg every 3–4 hr
Fentanyl (Duragesic)**	25-µg-per-hr patch	25-µg-per-hr patch
Patch	every 72 hr**	every 72 hr**
Hydrocodone (Vicodin, Lorcet+)		
Oral	NA‡	10 mg every 3–4 hr
Parenteral	NA	NA
Hydromorphone (Dilaudid)		
Oral	7.5mg every 3–4 hr	2–4 mg every 3–4 hr
Parenteral	1.5mg every 3–4 hr	1.5 mg every 3–4 hr
Levophanol (Levo-Dromoran)		
Oral	4 mg every 6–8 hr	4 mg every 6–8 hr
Parenteral	2 mg every 6–8 hr	2 mg every 6–8 hr
Meperidine (Demerol)		
Oral	300 mg every 2–3 hr	100 mg every 3 hr
Parenteral	100 mg every 3 hr	100 mg every 3 hr
Methadone (Dolophine)		
Oral	20 mg every 6–8 hr	5 mg every 8–12 hr
Parenteral	10 mg every 6–8 hr	5 mg every 8–12 hr
Morphine		
Oral	30 mg every 3–4 hr	15 mg every 3–4 hr
Parenteral	10 mg every 3–4 hr	10 mg every 3–4 hr
Morphine SR (MSContin)		
Oral	NA	15 mg every 8–12 hr
Parenteral	NA	NA
Oxycodone (Percocet, Perodan+)		
Oral	NA	15 mg every 3–4 hr
Parenteral	NA	NA
Oxycodone CR (OxyContin)		
Oral	NA	10 mg every 8–12 hr
Parenteral	NA	NA

* The information is adapted from Ballantyne, J., ed., *The Massachusetts General Handbook of Pain Management*, second ed., Philadelphia, PA: Lippincott, Williams & Wilkins, 2002: 562. Equivalent doses of opioids vary markedly according to source. A low dose of an opioid should be used to start and should be gradually increased until a dose is established that combines maximal analgesia with minimal adverse effects. A short-acting opioid should be used when the patient's pain is occasional, and a long-acting opioid when the pain is constant and frequent. A short-acting opioid can be added to a long-acting opioid to treat breakthrough or incidental pain, but in the treatment of chronic pain, the use of non-medical strategies to treat breakthrough pain is preferable. Rapid or frequent increases in dose should be avoided. Opioid rotation may be useful when dose escalation fails. The new opioid can be started at one-half to one-quarter of the calculated equivalent dose of the previously prescribed opioid.

NA denotes not applicable

** This is the lowest available dose. There is a risk of overdose in patients unaccustomed to opioid therapy.

+ These are combination formulations (with acetaminophen or aspirin), which have limited usefulness in the treatment of chronic pain.

APPENDIX B:
PAIN MANAGEMENT POLICY

PURPOSE:

The purpose of this policy is to state the Health System's commitment to provide a dignified, comprehensive, and collaborative approach to pain management consistent with the *Ethical and Religious Directives for Catholic Health Care.*

POLICY:

The Health System believes that patients have the right to maximal pain relief at all stages of their acute and/or chronic disease processes. We recognize that appropriate pain management is critical in the care of patients and believe that all patients are entitled to a dignified, comprehensive, and collaborative approach to pain management. While we realize that some medicines that alleviate pain in the dying patient may indirectly shorten the patient's life, our goal is to relieve pain and suffering as much as possible.

Although maximal pain relief is the right of all patients, some patients may choose to endure some aspects of their pain as an affirmation of their religious beliefs. The theological foundation of pain management for Christians is rooted in the passion of Christ. "Physical suffering is certainly an unavoidable element of the human condition. . . . According to Christian teaching, however, suffering, especially during the last moments of life, has a special place in God's saving plan; it is in fact a sharing in Christ's Passion and a union with the redeeming sacrifice which he offered in obedience to the father's will. Therefore, one must not be surprised if some Christians prefer to moderate their use of painkillers, in order to accept voluntarily at least part of their sufferings and thus associate themselves in a conscious way with the sufferings of Christ crucified (cf. Matthew 27:34)."[1]

Respect for the dignity of each patient creates a responsibility for the health care team to respect the free and informed decision by the patient to make medical treatment decisions, including the degree of pain relief desired. The emphasis of pain management should be on the prevention, evaluation, and relief of pain. Comprehensive pain management is a multidisciplinary and collaborative effort that must address physical, psychological, spiritual, and social effects of unrelieved pain.

PRINCIPLES FOR PAIN MANAGEMENT:

A. The dignity of the human person creates a responsibility for medical professionals to relieve maximally the pain and suffering of patients.

B. Pain management must be tailored to the specific patient's needs and situation and include a comprehensive assessment of pain and an evaluation of the effectiveness of treatment.

C. Patients who possess decision-making capacity are the decision makers for the course of their medical treatment, including the degree of pain relief desired. For patients who lack decision-making capacity, the appropriate surrogate, acting in a compassionate and ethical manner, should be the decision maker.

D. Consistent with our policy of informed consent, placebos should not be used in the assessment and management of pain. However, complementary treatment modalities may be used.

E. All patients will have pain addressed as part of the plan of care and will be taught that pain management is an essential part of treatment.

F. Discharge instructions will include information about pain as it pertains to the patient's individual situation. This will include the cause(s) of pain, recognizing precipitating and relieving factors, available methods of relief and how to use them (including the importance of safe and effective use of medications), and communication with the physician relating to pain and its management.

I. PROCEDURE: GENERAL PAIN MANAGEMENT FOR PATIENTS

A. ASSESSMENT

1. Each patient will be assessed by the nurse and the health care professional on admission for the presence/absence of pain.

2. Each patient will be reassessed for the presence/absence of pain prior to, during, and/or following any intervention that may cause pain.

3. Each patient will be assessed for his/her previous experiences with pain, and beliefs about and preferences for pain assessment.

4. Every patient will have pain addressed as part of the plan of care.

5. Every patient will be educated to inform the health care professionals when he/she experiences pain, recognizing that communication of unrelieved pain is essential in helping to manage its relief.

    a. The staff will utilize one of the available pain scales in assessing a patient's pain. The scale used will be determined by the patient's age and cognitive function.

    b. Staff will educate patients with regard to prevention of pain or reduction of pain rather than chasing and reducing pain once pain is established.

6. The patient will be assessed and reassessed for pain. The frequency of assessment and reassessment is based on how well each patient's pain is controlled.

7. Documentation will reflect assessment, reassessment, education, interventions, and patient outcomes.

B. INTERVENTION

1. Response to a patient's complaint of pain will be timely in an attempt to provide quick relief of pain.

2. If initial interventions are not effective to decrease the pain to a level acceptable to the patient, additional methods of pain relief will be sought. These may include other available pharmacological methods as well as nonpharmacological methods.

3. If pain relief is suboptimal, the physician will be notified.

4. Documentation will reflect additional interventions, reassessments, and patient outcomes.

C. PAIN MANAGEMENT TEAM CONSULTATION

1. For hospitalized patients, a Pain Management Consult is recommended in the following situations:

    a. For any patient admitted with intractable pain.

    b. For any patient experiencing increasing pain or decreasing relief of pain by current methods utilized.

    c. For any patient situation in which the physician desires assistance with pain management for his/her patient.

D. PATIENT EDUCATION

1. Patient education is tailored to address the patient's needs, values, abilities, and assessed readiness to learn.

2. The goal of patient education is to include the patient in the management of his/her pain.

3. Education on pain management includes:

    a. A general overview of the causes, a rating scale to communicate pain and effectiveness of interventions, and the use of a diary to record occurrences, intensity, treatment, and relief.

    b. Pharmacological management.

    c. Nonpharmacological management.

II. PROCEDURE / GENERAL PAIN MANAGEMENT FOR THE GERIATRIC PATIENT

1. The health care professionals caring for the geriatric patient recognize that the geriatric patient:

    a. May suffer from multiple, chronic, painful illnesses and may take several medications.

    b. Is at greater risk for drug–drug and drug–disease interactions.

    c. Presents unique problems when assessing for pain—these include physiological, psychological, religious, and cultural changes associated with aging.

    d. May believe that their pain cannot be relieved and are stoic in reporting their pain (especially among the elderly and frail elderly).

    e. May have cognitive impairment, delirium, and dementia as well as sensory   problems (visual and hearing impairment).

2. Health Care professionals will adjust their assessments for the geriatric patient to include observations for behavioral cues to pain such as restlessness, agitation, or facial grimacing, recognizing that the absence of such behaviors does not negate the presence of pain.

3. When appropriate, caregivers or family members will be included when assessment of pain is necessary and will be asked about pain history, interventions, and patient outcomes.

III. PROCEDURE / GENERAL PAIN MANAGEMENT FOR THE PEDIATRIC PATIENT

1. The health care professionals caring for the pediatric patient recognize that the pediatric patient:

   a. Determines pain by many factors including medical/surgical condition, developmental level, emotional and cognitive state, personal concerns, meaning of pain, family issues and attitudes, religion, culture, and environment.

   b. Requires frequent assessment/reassessment of the presence, amount, intensity, quality, and location of pain.

   c. Requires prevention or reduction of anticipated pain, and when prevention is not possible, needs prompt alleviation of pain.

   d. May require the use of a different format for measuring pain—such as a "faces" pain-rating scale, gestures, or quality of cry.

2. Health Care professionals will adjust their assessments for the pediatric patient to include knowledge of the growth and development level of each individual child.

3. The assessment of the child will include a pain history, an evaluation of diagnoses such as infection that could cause the pain or an increase in the pain, evaluation of the pain severity and location, as well as observation of the child and his or her response to the environment.

4. When appropriate, patients, caregivers, or other family members will be included when the assessment of a child's pain is necessary.

5. All interventions are tailored to the developmental level and personality of the child.

IV. PROCEDURE: GENERAL PAIN MANAGEMENT FOR THE DYING PATIENT

1. Dying patients who possess decision-making capacity are the decision makers for the course of their medical treatment, including the degree of pain relief desired in the final state of life.

2. It is incumbent on health care professionals to make every effort to relieve the pain and suffering of the dying patient even if this requires either intermittent or continued administration of progressively larger doses of opioids. The goal of treatment is to relieve pain and suffering to the fullest extent possible.

3. Dying patients should be assured the maximal possible comfort even in the face of impending death as heralded by falling blood pressure, declining rate of respiration, or altered level of consciousness.

4. A variety of means for pain relief, including what the patient believes is effective, should be used.

5. Establish a relationship of trust with the patient, so that the patient will not feel abandoned.

V. CONTINUOUS QUALITY IMPROVEMENT

The process of managing pain in outpatients and its effectiveness will be monitored, evaluated, and revised to continually improve outcomes.

Six:
Palliative Care and Hospice

"Death is not the ultimate tragedy of life. The ultimate tragedy is depersonalization—dying in an alien and sterile area, separated from the spiritual nourishment that comes from being able to reach out to a living hand, separated from a desire to experience the things that make life worth living, separated from hope."[1]

Traditionally, medical care has had two mutually exclusive goals: to cure disease and prolong life, or to provide comfort care. Given this dichotomy, the decision to focus on reducing suffering is made usually only after life-prolonging treatment has been ineffectual and death is imminent, usually within days or hours.[2] As a result, one of the best-kept secrets in a hospital today is palliative care and hospice care. We estimate that of the 2.4 million Americans who die each year, about 80 percent end their lives in hospitals attached to the latest advances in technology; only 300,000 die at home under hospice care.[3] The reasons why more people do not receive palliative or hospice care include the patient's fear of abandonment and the unknown, the family's denial of the inevitability of death of their loved one, and the physician's denial of medicine's limitations. Unless the options of palliative or hospice care are offered to patients, the fears that people have of dying—fear of dying alone and fear of dying in pain—will continue to make the dying process one that often lacks dignity and respect.

Palliative care comes from the Latin word *palliare* which means to cloak. It is a form of medical care or treatment that concentrates on reducing the severity of the symptoms of a disease or slowing the disease's progress rather than providing a cure. Occasionally, it can be used with a curative therapy, providing that the curative therapy will not cause additional morbidity. The goal is to relieve suffering and improve the quality of life for patients with advanced illnesses—and their families—through scientific knowledge and skills, including communication with patients and family members; management of pain and other symptoms; psychosocial, spiritual, and bereavement support; and coordination of an array of medical and social services.[4] The World Health Organization (WHO) in 1990 defined palliative care as "the active care of patients whose disease is not responsive to curative treatment." This definition stresses the terminal nature of the disease.[5]

Hospice care is viewed as part of the philosophy that we call palliative care. Hospice is a centuries-old idea coming from the Latin word *hospes* meaning guest. Originally, it referred to the offering of a place of shelter and rest or what we refer to as "hospitality" to weary and sick travelers on a long journey. Over the centuries, it developed into a philosophy of care that recognizes death as the final stage of life and seeks to enable patients to continue an alert, pain-free life and to manage other symptoms so that their last days may be spent with dignity and quality, surrounded by their loved ones. Hospice care, like palliative care, affirms life and neither hastens nor postpones death. The focus of hospice and palliative care is to treat the whole person rather than the disease; it emphasizes quality rather than quantity or length of life.[6] In addition, emphasis is placed not only on the well-being of the patient but also on the well-being of the family caregivers. Hospice personnel provide care for the patient and the family twenty-four hours a day, seven days a week.

The history of hospice and palliative care dates back to ancient times. Some say the first hospice experience appears in the New Testament with the parable of the Good Samaritan (Luke 10: 29–37). The Good Samaritan bandaged the wounds of the man beaten and lying along the roadside, then took him to the closest inn and paid to have the man ministered to by the innkeeper. Others believe the first recorded hospice opened in AD 475 in Syria—by Fabiola, a Roman woman and follower of St. Jerome—as a place of rest for the traveler, the sick, and the dying. During the next 1,500 years, hospices, provided care for those on a journey. In the nineteenth century, a religious order established hospices for the dying in Ireland and London.[7]

"Until the twentieth century, most people spent their last days at home, surrounded, cared for, and comforted by family and friends. That tradition faded as hospitals became places of healing in many Western countries."[8] The modern notion of hospice began in 1967 when Dr. Cicely Saunders founded St. Christopher's Hospice in London. She is regarded as the founder of the modern hospice movement. As a physician, Saunders dedicated her life to the care of the dying and planned a model hospice that would provide exemplary palliative care and would incorporate teaching and research programs. She avowed the regular giving of strong narcotics, including heroin and the Brompron cocktail mixture of morphine and gin, as the proper regimen to ensure that a pain-free patient could maintain quality of life in the last days. St. Christopher's Hospice demonstrated the superior reliability and efficacy of oral morphine over heroin and reported the absence of tolerance and addiction in cancer patients, even with long-term use.[9]

The hospice movement in the United States began in the 1960s, but the first hospice to provide services was the Connecticut Hospice in March 1974. "In 1982, Congress created the Medicare hospice benefit, reserving such services for terminally ill Medicare beneficiaries with life expectancies of six months or less 'if the disease runs its normal course.' Effective with the enactment of the Balanced Budget Act of 1997, the Medicare hospice benefit was divided into the following benefit periods: (1) an initial 90-day period; (2) a subsequent 90-day period; and (3) an unlimited number of subsequent 60-day benefit periods as long as the patient continued to meet program eligibility requirements. Beneficiaries must be recertified as terminally ill at the beginning of each benefit period."[10] The relatively generous Medicare reimbursement for hospice treatment has increased hospice usage in the United States. The 1989 Congressional mandate increased reimbursement rates by 20 percent and tied future increases to the annual increase in the hospital market basket.

From 1984 to January 2006, the total number of hospices participating in Medicare rose from 31 to 2,884—a more than ninefold increase (see Appendix A). Of these, 1,648 are freestanding, 672 are home-health-agency-based, 551 are hospital-based, and 13 are skilled-nursing-facility-based.[11] The first hospital-based palliative care program in the United States began in 1989 at the Cleveland Clinic in response to the recognition that restrictions on hospice eligibility imposed by the Medicare hospice benefit prevented adequate care for seriously ill and dying patients in acute-care hospitals. In response, there has been a dramatic increase in hospital-based palliative care programs, now numbering more than 1,200.[12]

Hospice programs provide services in various settings: the home, hospice centers, hospitals, or skilled-nursing facilities. The number of hospice programs in the United States has continued to increase from the first program in 1974 to more than 4,100 programs today. The majority of the growth is in small free-standing programs, and 93 percent of agencies reported that they are Medicare certified. Nearly three out of four hospice programs are accredited by the Joint Commission on Accreditation of Health Care Organizations (JCAHO), the Community Health Accreditation Program (CHAP), the Accreditation Commission for Health Care (ACHC), or another accrediting agency. Fully 67.6 percent of programs reported non-profit (501c3) status, while 27.2 percent reported for-profit status. Government-run programs account for 5.2 percent of all programs.[13]

The criteria for hospice care under the Medicare benefit require that patients acknowledge they are in the dying process and are willing to forego insurance coverage for life-prolonging treatments, and that two physicians certify that the patient has a life expectancy of six months or less. Studies have shown that referral to palliative-care programs and hospice results in beneficial effects on patients' symptoms, reduced hospital costs, greater likelihood of death at home, and a higher level of patient and family satisfaction than does conventional care.[14]

The principles that constitute the National Hospice Organization's "Philosophy of Hospice" are these:

1. Hospice implies acceptance of death as a natural part of the cycle of life.
2. When death is inevitable, hospice will neither seek to hasten it nor to postpone it.
3. Patients, their families, and loved ones are the unit of care.
4. Psychological pain and spiritual pain are as significant as physical pain, and addressing all three requires the skills and approach of an interdisciplinary team.
5. Pain relief and symptom control are appropriate clinical goals; the goal of all intervention is to maximize the quality of remaining life through the provision of palliative therapies.
6. Care is provided regardless of ability to pay.[15]

The principles of hospice and palliative care are based on a shift in the patient's treatment from curative to palliative care. This shift rarely takes place at a specific moment. "Just as the disease treatment is a process, so too is preparing a patient for the time when treatment for cure is no longer an option. Preparing a patient begins with an honest discussion of the disease and its outcomes."[16] Physicians have the ethical responsibility to be honest with their patients about their medical condition. When there are no further treatments to cure the disease, the patient must be informed of this fact but must also be given the option of palliative care and hospice care as a treatment. "Presenting hospice as a medical option for treating a terminal illness can help with many unknowns—'fears of uncontrollable pain, nausea, vomiting, embarrassment, and especially abandonment' that often accompany end-stage diseases."[17]

The focus of hospice is to provide services to patients *and* their families to assist and support them during the dying process. The family of the patient and others involved with the patient can be crucial in any hospice discussion and care plan. In many cases, the patient may be ready to accept hospice care but family members and friends are not. At times, they can even coerce the patient into continuing aggressive treatment even though the burdens outweigh the benefits. That is why the family should be included in these discussions whenever possible but always with the patient's consent. Many times all the family needs to hear is that the patient has accepted the diagnosis of the terminal condition and that it is his or her choice to accept hospice care.[18] Hospice treats the patient and the family as a unit and unless both parties understand the principles and the goal of hospice, the services offered will fail to be beneficial to all parties concerned.

Hospice services are offered by a multidisciplinary team whose emphasis is on maximizing comfort for the terminally ill patient and supporting the family members and other loved ones. The hospice team consists of physicians, nurses, health care aides, spiritual counselors, social workers, volunteers, ancillary therapists, and bereavement counselors. The services offered by the hospice team include pain and symptom relief, spiritual care, home care and inpatient care, respite care, family conferences, and bereavement care. (Examples can be found in Appendixes B, C, D, and E.) The services offered are extensive and wide-ranging. For example, hospice care integrates complementary therapies with conventional care such as relaxation therapy, massage therapy, music therapy, and acupuncture to relieve symptoms and other causes of pain. Trained bereavement counselors offer support and guidance for patients and family members. This support continues for up to a year after the death of the patient. The most common concerns found among those in a terminal condition are fear of pain, loss of independence, worries about family, and feeling like a burden. The hospice team provides comprehensive palliative care aimed at relieving symptoms, treating depression in patients, and giving social, emotional, and spiritual support to both the patient and the family.

Despite these services, only 1.2 million patients received services from hospices in 2005, an increase of more than 150,000 people over the previous year. In 2005, approximately one-third of all deaths in the United

States were under the care of a hospice program. The 1.2 million hospice patients served includes about 800,000 who died, 200,000 who were admitted in 2005 but carried over to 2006, and 200,000 who were discharged alive. According to specialists in the field, however, perhaps twice as many patients should have been in hospice programs. Four out of five hospice patients are 65 years of age or older, while one-third of all hospice patients are 85 years of age or older. Pediatric patients account for less than 1 percent of patients. Almost as many males as females are hospice patients and most are married. The most common terminal illness among hospice patients is cancer.[19]

In the last decade, about forty perinatal hospice programs have been started in the United States. Perinatal hospices are for those families who give birth to babies with fatal anomalies. Statistics show that 20 to 40 percent of parents given a diagnosis of a fatal fetal condition do not opt to abort the fetus but to carry the fetus to term. Perinatal hospices help families gain control over an event that could be devastating. In general, parents allow these babies to die without aggressive medical intervention such as feeding tubes, intravenous fluids, and surgeries. They allow for medications to ease the child's discomfort. Most of these children die within hours of birth, but about 30 percent go home with their families where they eventually die.[20]

In 2006, the average length of hospice service increased from 57 to 59 days. The median length of stay also increased from 22 to 25 days. Although the length of stay is increasing, many of those who entered hospice care did so only at the very end of their illnesses, spending a week or less in a program that ideally would have helped them cope with the final six months or year of life.[21] Very little comfort and support can be given to patients and family members in such a short period of time. This is frustrating not only for the patient and family but also for the hospice personnel.

Another interesting statistic is that fewer than two in ten patients admitted to hospice care are minorities—84 percent are white, 8 percent are African American, and 8 percent are from other minorities. The percentage of minority patients rose from 16.5 percent in 2004 to 17.8 percent in 2005. There are many reasons for the low number of minorities in hospice. They might harbor a mistrust of the medical profession (dating back to the historical atrocities when Black Americans were denied adequate health care or were used as experimental subjects without their knowledge in the Tuskegee Syphilis Study)[22] they might not want strangers in their homes; they might have spiritual traditions that hold that God, not a doctor, determines who lives and who dies; and they might hold more firmly to a belief in miracles.

Many African Americans will opt to die in a hospital because they believe that only there will they get all the treatment the medical profession has to offer (like the whites receive). This is why African Americans and other minorities are less likely than whites to consent to DNR orders or to write advance directives or living wills. Much of the research on ethnic and racial influences on end-of-life decision making is based on anecdotal information. What is needed is evidence-based research so that recommendations can be made to develop strategies for integrating ethnicity-specific components into end-of-life care.[23] Unless something is done to overcome these suspicions, African Americans and other minorities will continue to receive less palliative care at the end of life.

National health care expenditures for 2006 are projected at $2,163.9 billion. The percentage of patients covered by the Medicare hospice benefit (versus other payment sources) increased to 82.4% in 2005.This increase is likely due to having more complete payer mix data from several states. A decline was seen in the percentage of patients covered by Medicaid, self-payment, and charity care.[24] In addition to Medicare and Medicaid funding, the other sources of hospice revenue are private insurance companies, community donations, and grants. Medicare hospice expenditures climbed from $205.4 million in 1989 to more than $6.7 billion in 2004, but the Medicare hospice benefit still represents a small portion of the total Medicare spending. In 2005, an estimated 2.5 percent of Medicare benefit payments were spent on hospice care. The projections in 2006 show that hospice care will continue to be a small part of total Medicare spending. Approximately 43% of the estimated $331 billion in Medicare spending for 2005 and 36 percent of the projected $390 billion in spending in 2006 will go to hospitals. In 2005, approximately 17 percent of Medicare spending will go to physician services—approximately 15 percent in 2006[25] (see Appendix F).

The Hospice Association of America estimates that Medicare reimbursements for routine home care is $126.49 a day; continuous home care day is $738.26 for 24 hours or $30.76 per hour; inpatient respite care day is $130.85; and general inpatient care provided in a Medicare-certified hospital, skilled nursing facility, or inpatient unit of hospice is $562.69 a day.[26] It is believed that due to our aging population, an increasing interest and concern for end-of-life care, and rising health care costs, the need for Medicare-certified hospices will continue to grow.[27] Despite these costs, hospice care is still more cost-effective than hospital and skilled nursing care facilities. There have been various studies on the cost-effectiveness of hospice care, both federally and privately sponsored, which provide strong evidence that hospice is a less costly approach to care for the terminally ill (see Appendix F).[28]

One of the biggest deterrents for individuals regarding hospice is that most individuals with a terminal condition who wish to enter hospice care must forego advanced medical treatment to qualify for hospice care. This means cancer patients, under most circumstances unless it is for palliative care, must pass up chemotherapy, and patients with kidney failure must abandon dialysis. This either–or decision has caused some patients who would greatly benefit from hospice care to opt for aggressive in-hospital treatments, which are far more costly.

Recently, some hospice programs and private health insurers have initiated a new approach called "open access" to encourage patients to get on hospice for their last months of life. This new approach allows hospice programs to offer advanced medical treatment even when they are not paid more to do so. Proponents argue that it is an example of the efforts of some insurers and health care providers to try to fix specific problems in the nation's medical system. Aetna and United Health are allowing some patients to have potentially life-prolonging medical treatment while on hospice. Physicians argue that the either–or approach is less valid today in that continued advances in medicine are allowing even patients with very advanced diseases to benefit from new treatments. The Aetna experiment allows 40,000 of its roughly 15 million insured members to be eligible for these services. The initial results have shown that people will take advantage of hospice care if they do not have to give up other treatments to prolong their lives. In the long run, this will be cost-effective and it allows patients more time to take advantage of hospice benefits.

The Aetna experiment is the exception, and Medicare still requires patients to give up regular medical coverage if they enter the hospice program. Opponents argue that this experiment is misguided because it causes patients to spend their last days in a hospital receiving expensive care that may not even be beneficial. Many hospice programs are too small to spread their costs, which would allow them to take patients needing expensive treatments. Some are arguing that Medicare should drop its requirement that patients forego other coverage if they want hospice care. Senator Ron Wyden of Oregon has introduced legislation that would end the Medicare requirement. He argues that the change would not significantly raise

Medicare spending, but that it would give people more control over the way they die. Aetna plans to continue this experiment, because in the first year the average length of stay in hospice increased to 34 days—up from 27 days. Aetna may in fact end up extending its coverage to more of its insured members.[29]

Most hospices are run by nonprofit, independent organizations. Some are affiliated with hospitals, nursing homes, or home health care agencies, and there are some that are for-profit organizations. Determining which hospice would be best for a patient may take some research. Most patients and families hear about hospice from their physician, nurse, or social worker. One can also find information about hospices from the National Hospice and Palliative Care Organization (http://www.nhpco.org/templates/1/homepage.cfm), state hospice organizations, or the state health department. The telephone number for state hospice organizations and health departments can be found in the state government section of the local telephone directory.

The Medicare hotline can also answer general questions about Medicare benefits and coverage and can refer people to their regional home health intermediary for information about Medicare-certified hospice programs. The toll-free telephone number is 1-800-MEDICARE (1-800-633-4227). Deaf and hearing impaired callers with TTY equipment can call 1-877-486-2048. The booklet *Medicare Hospice Benefits* is the official publication for Medicare hospice benefits. The booklet, which outlines the type of hospice care under Medicare and provides detailed information about hospice coverage, is available at http://www.medicare.gov/Publications/Pubs/pdf/02154.pdf on the Internet. Information about Medicaid benefits can be accessed at http://cms.hhs.gov/medicaid on the Internet.[30]

It is recommended that when evaluating hospice programs the following questions should be addressed:

1. Is the hospice Medicare-certified?
2. What services are available to the patient?
3. What services are offered to the family?
4. What bereavement services are available?
5. How involved are the family members?
6. How involved is the doctor?
7. Who makes up the hospice care team, and how are they trained and screened?
8. How will the individual's pain and symptoms be managed?

9. If circumstances change, can services be provided in different settings? Does the hospice have contacts with local nursing homes? Is residential hospice available?

10. Is the program reviewed and licensed by the state or certified in some other way?

11. Are all costs covered by insurance?[31]

Finding the right hospice for a patient is essential. It is important that patients and family members examine the available options and select the hospice that is the most advantageous for the particular individual in his or her condition.

The general consensus is that hospice care is very beneficial for both patients and family members, but it is not without its critics. Felicia Ackerman argues that some of the principles of hospice care depend on a highly questionable ideology that, while valuable to some terminally ill patients, can be reasonably rejected by others. She uses as an example the fact that hospice is not religiously based, but she agrees that it does seem to have a religious foundation. Although serenity in the face of impending death is reasonable for those who are confident of the afterlife, she asks why those individuals who believe their death will be the unequivocal and permanent end of their existence should expect such serenity. Ackerman questions whether such expectations constitute an attempt to export religion-based attitudes.[32]

Ackerman also argues that "when its principles are fully scrutinized and understood, hospice care will be seen, not as 'the most effective route to a dignified death,' but as just one option for the terminally ill, whose other options should include experimental attempts at a cure, high-tech life-prolongation, and perhaps even assisted suicide."[33] This position is based on giving all terminally ill patients the right to choose any option of treatment. What Ackerman fails to consider is that some of these options are neither in the best interest of the patient nor in the best interest of society as a whole. Medical resources are limited and using these resources on patients who will not benefit from them violates both the ethical principle of beneficence and the principle of justice (because this is not a just allocation of resources).

Despite all the services that hospice offers to patients and families, it is still one of the best-kept secrets in hospitals and nursing homes. There are many reasons for this, ranging from the patient's fear of accepting death, to the family's pressure on the patient not to give up hope, and the physician's denial that there is nothing more that can be done for the patient clinically. However, there seems to be a trend in the United States, and as more patients and families become educated about the benefits of hospice and palliative care, it is becoming a more attractive option than dying in a hospital attached to the latest advances in technology.

Hospitals and nursing homes need to initiate palliative care policies not only to benefit patients but to encourage physicians, nurses, and social workers to make palliative and hospice care a priority for all terminally ill patients. (For a sample palliative care policy, see Appendix G.) For hospice and palliative care to become a more valuable option for the terminally ill, physicians, nurses, and social workers need to initiate conversations about the benefits of these programs at the appropriate time. When a patient has been diagnosed with a terminal condition and further medical treatment would appear not to be beneficial, that is the time to begin the conversation. Patients and family members often need time to digest the fact that the disease process has advanced, and the patient's basic needs have changed from a curative mode of care to a palliative mode.

Besides initiating such a conversation, physicians also need to take the time to listen to patients and their loved ones so that they truly comprehend how much the patient and family members understand and what the values are that form their decision making. Physicians need to help patients walk their final journey with dignity, peace, and compassion—supporting their loved ones throughout the process.[34] Recent studies have shown "lower morbidity and mortality and better emotional support among surviving family members of hospice patients than among family members of patients who did not receive hospice services, although it is uncertain whether this difference reflects the nature of families who elect hospice care rather than the effects of the intervention."[35]

The advantages of hospice and palliative care have been shown to benefit not only patients and family members but also society as a whole. Until health care professionals, patients, and families become more comfortable talking about the death and dying process, the fear is that hospice and palliative care, excellent options for accessing supportive services during an extremely difficult time, will remain marginalized.[36] Hospice and palliative care can no longer be viewed as abandonment and giving up hope. Instead, they must be seen as providing the care that the patient and the family need and deserve.

Appendix A:
Number of Medicare-certified Hospices and Program Payments, by State, 2004

State	Number of Hospices	Number of Persons	Number of Hospice Days	Program Payments ($ thousands)
AL	103	22,558	2,299,041	251,916
AK	3	221	15,263	2,215
AZ	44	24,104	1,693,943	236,889
AR	47	7,952	571,955	63,221
CA	181	72,437	4,179,191	621,041
CO	41	12,475	746,898	100,932
CT	26	7,468	346,497	56,833
DE	6	2,331	133,165	17,806
DC	2	805	33,328	4,999
FL	41	81,432	5,203,856	795,302
GA	87	23,076	1,601,918	206,138
HI	7	1,765	84,330	13,397
ID	27	3,272	198,673	23,665
IL	95	31,489	1,633,034	230,337
IN	76	17,789	1,187,375	147,565
IA	65	10,527	581,688	66,997
KS	48	7,442	538,063	59,183
KY	27	10,515	619,755	78,113
LA	71	12,746	798,024	95,460
ME	18	2,745	161,552	19,980
MD	27	10,789	490,684	64,973
MA	45	15,285	797,986	118,057
MI	85	31,438	1,595,307	208,085
MN	60	11,273	656,659	87,194
MS	72	12,533	1,440,067	157,310
MO	78	20,735	1,458,417	150,642
MT	24	2,160	118,178	14,059
NE	30	4,459	222,665	26,493
NV	11	6,462	368,352	59,410
NH	19	2,557	115,794	17,335
NJ	46	20,394	1,013,475	144,063

NM	38	6,044	506,220	61,720
NY	52	30,713	1,532,582	231,956
NC	80	22,476	1,546,303	196,330
ND	15	1,485	81,043	9,523
OH	91	39,400	2,151,654	295,336
OK	125	18,293	1,910,607	207,895
OR	44	13,003	1,100,088	87,263
PA	129	40,837	2,102,061	270,292
PR	34	6,589	650,148	51,454
RI	8	2,995	133,104	20,595
SC	45	10,943	790,826	94,643
SD	15	1,489	60,872	7,285
TN	50	14,238	836,694	105,805
TX	191	58,673	3,980,362	509,670
UT	40	7,417	764,075	77,399
VT	10	1,072	52,740	6,502
VI	1	71	7,259	849
VA	57	14,638	817,972	100,944
WA	31	13,976	690,575	96,513
WV	19	4,929	308,773	36,548
WI	51	14,684	801,273	104,178
WY	18	668	40,653	4,971

Source: Centers for Medicare & Medicaid Services, Health Care Information System (HCIS), October 2005.

Notes: Medicare program payments represent fee-for-service only—that is, program payments exclude amounts paid for managed care services. State column includes District of Columbia, Puerto Rico, and the U.S. Virgin Islands. Numbers may not add to totals because of rounding.

Appendix B:
General Guidelines When Taking Medications

1. Always read directions on the label carefully. Contact your nurse or pharmacist for clarification if you have any questions.

2. Do not mix different medications in one container. Keep medicine in original container with label from the pharmacy.

3. Do not store medicines for long periods of time. Most should be discarded after 6 months if not in use.

4. Do not stop taking any medication without first consulting with your doctor or nurse, unless a specific time limit was given when the medication was ordered.

5. On the Hospice medication information forms, some abbreviations are used:

BM	=	bowel movement
GI	=	gastrointestinal
N/V	=	nausea, vomiting
N/V/D	=	nausea, vomiting, diarrhea
W/	=	with

6. Many patients experience no side effects(s), but all medications have the potential for producing some degree of side effect(s), which can be experienced in varying degrees. If a side effect is pronounced or very uncomfortable, report this to your nurse or physician.

7. Some medications do not absorb well if there is food or antacids in the stomach and must be taken on an empty stomach. **Read the label carefully.** Contact your nurse or pharmacist if the direction is unclear.

8.   DO NOT cut, crush, or dissolve medications without checking with your nurse or pharmacist. If you have difficulty swallowing, a medication may be available in liquid form. Contact your nurse.

9.   Be sure to let your nurse know if you are taking any nonprescription medication such as Tylenol or Aspirin.

10.   Wash your hands before and after handling medications.

11.   Wear gloves when administering suppositories or creams.

12.   Don't store medications in a moist area such as the bathroom.

13.   Prescription Refill Information
You may call the pharmacy to arrange for prescription refills provided that there are refills left on the prescription.

   ▪   Check the label on the bottle to make sure you have refills available.
   ▪   Give the prescription number for the medication(s) that you want the pharmacy to refill.

If you do not have any refills left on your prescription, you will need to contact the hospice nurse or your physician to arrange for a medication renewal.

Please, do not allow yourself to run out of medication—especially heading into a weekend or holiday. We recommend that you get into a routine or habit of checking all medications on Thursdays to make sure you have enough. This allows for sufficient time to contact the doctor, if needed, before the weekend.

14.   Dispose of all unused controlled substances only in the presence of he hospice nurse when the patient no longer requires such medications.

Appendix C:
What to Do When Breathing Is Very Difficult:

ELEVATE THE HEAD
An upright position is best. Raise the head of the bed, or sit in a chair.

USE A FAN
Place a fan so that it is directed to blow on the face, across the cheeks.

USE OXYGEN
Oxygen by nasal tips can be used at one to three liters per minute. Use the oxygen as long as needed. When you begin to feel more comfortable, you may decrease the flow rate to one or two or remove the oxygen for brief periods. If your nose becomes dry, use K-Y jelly to lubricate it or ask your nurse for suggestions.
DO NOT USE VASELINE or petrolatum Products.

Your doctor may order a different flow rate.
The nurse will write in this flow rate:_____

If you do not have oxygen, CALL THE HOSPICE NURSE ANY TIME OF NIGHT OR DAY. While waiting for delivery, keep your head elevated, use a fan, and ask someone to sit with you. Try to minimize activity and exertion.

USE MEDICATIONS
1. Roxanol
Enhances relaxation/rest and relieves the sense of difficult breathing. Can be mixed with a small amount of juice or water if too bitter. If there is difficulty swallowing, or it produces nausea, it can be placed under the tongue.

2. Nebulizer treatment

   The medication is placed in the small jar and the "Neb machine" creates a mist. As you hold the mouthpiece and breathe in your usual way, the medicated mist travels into the airway passages, opening them. Treatment time is approximately ten minutes. This helps to relieve congestion and wheezing.

   Your nurse will write in any other instructions:

   _____

   _____

   _____

APPENDIX D:

COORDINATION OF CARE FOR EARLY, MIDDLE, AND LATE STAGES OF SERIOUS CHRONIC ILLNESSES. *

PALLIATIVE CARE SERVICES	EARLY STAGE	MIDDLE STAGE	LATE STAGE
Goals of care	Discuss diagnosis, prognosis, likely course of the illness, and disease-modifying therapies; talk about patient-centered goals, hopes, and expectations for medical treatments.	Review patient's understanding of prognosis; review efficacy and benefit-to-burden ratio for disease-modifying treatments; re-assess goals of care and expectations; prepare patient and patient's family for a shift in goals; encourage paying attention to important tasks, relationships, and financial affairs.	Assess patient's understanding of diagnosis, disease course, and prognosis; review appropriateness of disease-goals of care and recommend appropriate shifts; help patient explicitly plan for a peaceful death; encourage completion of important task increased attention to relationships and financial affairs.
Programmatic support	Advise patient to sign up for visiting nurse and home care services and case-management services (if available).	Advise patient to sign up for visiting nurse and home care services; consider palliative care program in hospital or at home, hospice, subacute rehabilitation case-management services, and PACE.	Advise patient to sign up for palliative care program in hospital or at home, case-management services, hospice, PACE; consider nursing home placement with hospice or palliative care if patient's home caregivers are overwhelmed.

	Early stage	Middle stage	Late stage
Financial Planning	Advise patient to seek help in planning for financial, long-term care, and insurance needs and to begin transfer of assets if patient is considering a future Medicaid application, refer patient to a lawyer who is experienced in health issues.	Advise patient to reassess adequacy of planning for financial, medical, home care, prescription, long-term care, and family-support needs; consider hospice referral and Medicaid eligibility	Advise patient to review all financial resources and needs; inform patient and family about financial options for personal and long-term care (e.g., hospice and Medicaid) if resources are inadequate to meet needs; explicitly recommend hospice and review its advantages; consider Medicaid eligibility.
Family support	Inform patient and family about support groups; ask about practical support needs (e.g., transportation, prescription-drug coverage, respite care, and personal care); listen to concerns.	Encourage support or counseling for family caregivers; ensure that caregivers have information about practical resources, stress depression and adequacy of medical care; identify respite and practical support Resources; recommend help from friends; raise the possibility of hospice and discuss it benefits.	Encourage out-of-town family to visit; refer caregivers to disease-specific support groups or counseling inquire routinely about health, well-being, and practical needs of caregivers; offer resources for respite care; after death, send bereavement card and call after patient's death; listen to concerns.

*Early stage refers to the stage of disease at the time of diagnosis, middle stage to progressive disease and increasing functional decline, and late stage to the stage when death is imminent. PACE denotes Program of All-Inclusive Care for the Elderly.

APPENDIX E:
FOOD–DRUG INTERACTION SHEET

DRUG NAME	RECOMMENDATION	REASON
1. Captopril (Capoten)	Take 1 hour before or 2 hours after a meal.	Eating can lower (↓) drugs effect.
2. Cipro (Cirpofloxacin)	Avoid taking large amounts of drinks with caffeine like coffee, tea, some drinks (Mello Yello, Mountain Dew, Kick, Colas, Dr. Pepper, Mr. PIBB) and chocolate Products.	This drug with caffeine can make you more nervous, unable to sleep and have a fast heart beat.
3. Didanosine (Videx, ddi)	Take on an empty stomach Drug should be taken 1 or 2 hours after a meal is eaten. If taken too close to a meal, take with an antacid. Tablets should not be swallowed whole. They are to be chewed well or crushed and mixed with at least an ounce of water.	Food in the stomach will lower how drug works.
4. Flagyl (Metronidazole)	Take with food avoid alcohol (including cough syrups with alcohol. Do not consume alcohol for at least one full day after drug is stopped.	Taking with food will lower (↓) stomach upset. Use of alcohol may cause a fast heart beat, chest pains, flushing.

Drug Name	Recommendation	Reason
5. Indinavir (Crixivan)	Take on an empty stomach 1hour before or 2 hours after a meal or take with low-fat, low protein snack. Drink at least six (8oz.) glasses of water every day.	High fat /high protein foods can lower how well the drug work. Drinking (8 oz.) glasses of water may help to lower the chance of forming a kidney stone by "flushing" the drug through the kidneys.
6. Monoamine Oxidase Inhibitors Phenelzine (Nardil) Tranlcypromine (Parnate)	Avoid foods and drinks with tyramine or tryptophan while taking MAOI's and for 2 weeks after stopping this drug. These Foods and drinks include alcoholic Beverages, especially wine (Chianti and Champagne) and beer; alcohol-free beer, cheeses (strong aged or processed types); bananas; raisins; sour cream, yogurt; pickled herring; (chicken liver) dry sausage (including hard salami and pepperoni); canned figs; avocados; soy sauce; yeast extracts; papaya products including certain meat tenderizers; fava beans; and broad bean pods. Large amounts of caffeine and chocolate should be avoided as well.	Eating tyramine or tryptophan foods can cause fatal increase(↑)in blood pressure. Symptoms include severe headache, neck stiffness and soreness, nausea/ vomiting, sweating, visual changes, chest pain and changes in heart rate.

Drug Name	Recommendation	Reason
7. Phenytoin Suspensions (Dilantin) & Tube Feeding	Hold tube feeding for 1 hour before and 1 hour after taking Dilantin suspension.	Tube feedings lower (↓) Dilantin's effect.
8. Tetracycline (Sumycin, Achromycin Panmycin)	Take 1hour before or 2 hours after a meal or dairy food. Avoid use of tetracyclines with antacids, laxatives, dairy products or iron pills If an antacid must be taken, take 2-3 hours before or after tetracycline. Take with a full glass of water.	Drinking a full glass of water can avoid stomach upset. Taking with food, milk or antacids can lower drug effect.
9. Warfarin(Coumadin)	Eat a steady amount of food containing Vit. K. include: soybean oil, beef liver, chicken liver, port liver, green tea, leaves, spinach, green tomato, turnip greens. You do not have to avoid these foods. Consult doctor or dietitian before making major diet changes.	Changes in the amount of Vit. K you eat may affect the way the drug works. Eating too much or too little Vit. K. will affect how fast your blood will clot.

APPENDIX F:
COMPARISON OF HOSPITAL, SNF, AND HOSPICE MEDICARE CHARGES, 1998-2005

	1998	1999	2000	2001	2002	2003	2004	2005
Hospital inpatient charges per day	$2,177	$2,583	$2,762	$3,069	$3,574	$4,117	$4,559	$4,787
Skilled nursing facilitycharges per day	482	424	413	422	475	487	493	521
Hospice charges per covered day of care	113	113	118	120	125	126	129	131

Sources: The hospital and SNF Medicare charge data are from the Annual Statistical Supplement, 2005, to the Social security bulletin, Social security Administration. Hospital and SNF data for 2005 are updated using the Bureau of Labor statistics' (BLS) Hospital Producer Price Index (PPI) and the BLS Nursing Care Facility PPI, respectively. The hospice charge data for 1998 are from the Health Care Financing Review (HCFR), Statistical Supplement, Health Care Financing Administration, 2000. Hospice data for 1999 are from the HCFR, Statistical Supplement.

Appendix G:
Sample Palliative Care Policy

Purpose

The purposes of this policy are these:

- To clarify the meaning of palliative care, often referred to as "comfort care."

- To promote comprehensive and consistent palliative care.

- To establish a process for determining appropriate palliative care for individual patients.

Policy

The Health System recognizes that in the care of patients with advanced disease it is medically appropriate and ethically acceptable to shift the primary goal of treatment to palliative care if this is judged to be medically appropriate by the patient's physician and consistent with the wishes of the patient or the patient's surrogate.

I. Definition

Palliative care consists of all treatments and services aimed at alleviating physical symptoms and addressing the psychological, social, and spiritual needs of the patients and their families so as to enhance patients' and families' quality of life to the greatest degree possible.

Palliative Care:

- affirms life and regards dying as a normal process;

- implies the cessation of all diagnostic measures and all life-sustaining and other therapeutic treatments that do not directly contribute to the patient's comfort or to patient and family goals;

- consists of active management of pain and other distressing symptoms (In the relief of pain, it is ethically permissible to ad-

173

minister analgesics, in sufficient amounts, to control the patient's pain, even if this has the unintended effect of depressing the patient's respiratory function.); and

- is multidisciplinary in order to address the physical, psychosocial and spiritual needs of patient and family.

II. Procedure

A. A discussion should be initiated between the attending physician and the patient and/or the patient's family about the appropriateness of shifting goals of treatment to palliative care.

B. The attending physician and other members of the health care team should develop a palliative care plan with the patient and/or the patient's family (usually in the context of a family conference), taking into account their particular goals and needs. Special attention should be given to:

- what therapies and procedures should be continued, discontinued, or initiated;
- symptom control, especially the management of pain and anxiety;
- the most appropriate setting for the patient's death, including the appropriateness of hospice care.

C. The physician should document the patient's and/or family's agreement with the plan in the medical record.

D. The physician should complete the "Palliative Care Order Form." A general order like "comfort care only" is not acceptable.

E. A regular review of the palliative care plan should occur and adjustments should be made as the patient's condition changes.

ADULT PALLIATIVE CARE ORDER FORM

DATE: _____
TIME: _____

1.   RESUSCITATION STATUS
     This patient is no-CPR. In the event of cardiac or respiratory arrest, cardiopulmonary resuscitation will not be attempted. No "code blue" should be called.

2.   INITIATE THE FOLLOWING ORDERS TO PROVIDE COMFORT:

Pain/air hunger: _____

Anxiety/delirium: _____

Sleep: _____

Constipation: _____

Diarrhea: _____

Nausea/vomiting: _____

Thirst:_____

Fever: _____

Other:_____

3.   The following therapies may not contribute to providing comfort. If this patient is currently receiving any of these, please indicate below if they
are to be continued or discontinued.

IV hydration	Continue	Discontinue
Diagnostic procedures	Continue	Discontinue
ECG and O2 sat monitoring	Continue	Discontinue
Supplemental O2	Continue	Discontinue
Parenteral and/or enteral nutrition	Continue	Discontinue
Arterial lines	Continue	Discontinue
Central venous lines	Continue	Discontinue
Peripheral venous lines	Continue	Discontinue
PT/OT	Continue	Discontinue
Blood products	Continue	Discontinue
Radiation therapy	Continue	Discontinue
Dialysis (Please notify nephrologist, Dr. _____)	Continue	Discontinue
Blood draws for standing laboratory orders	Continue	Discontinue

4.   Please discontinue the following medications:

_____

5.   Consult Pastoral Care and Social Work Departments.

6.   Hospice Department to evaluate patient for appropriateness of hospice care.

Transfer orders:

_____

SEVEN:
SPIRITUALITY AND END-OF-LIFE CARE

There has been an ongoing debate in medicine for centuries about whether there is a relationship between spirituality and health—or, more specifically, between spirituality and end-of-life care. Countless studies have been done on this topic, but there is still not a definitive answer. Maybe this is one of those questions in life that one has to answer for oneself. As patients and their families confront diseases such as cancer, Parkinson's, Alzheimer's, or HIV/AIDS, they are confronted with decisions about whether, at the end-stage of their disease, they should continue to seek aggressive treatment. Or would it be more appropriate to accept the inevitable and move toward palliative care. Questions arise about experimental treatments, additional rounds of chemotherapy, further surgeries, tube feedings, and mechanical ventilation—all for the purpose of extending life. Issues about quality of life, quality of function, dignity, and respect seem to be pushed to the sidelines by the emphasis on quantity—rather than quality—of life.

The prophet Isaiah writes: "Why spend your money for what is not bread; your wages for what fails to satisfy?" (Isaiah 55:2). One might wonder if he was not talking about extraordinary end-of-life treatments. Death is inevitable and the Judeo-Christian tradition has always attempted to walk a balanced middle path between medical vitalism (that aims to preserve life at any cost) and medical pessimism (that kills when life seems frustrating, burdensome, or "useless"). Both of these extremes are rooted in an identical idolatry of life—an attitude that, at least by inference, views death as an unmitigated, absolute evil, and life as the absolute good.[1]

Just because we have the technological ability to extend life does not mean it should always be done. It is at this point that the patient reaches a crossroads. Does the patient continue aggressive treatment that in reality is nonbenficial, or does the patient accept the inevitable and move toward comfort measures? It is at this moment, when the patient is confronted with his or her own mortality, that spiritual and religious concerns can become awakened or intensified. These religious and spiritual values are often the basis for a patient's decision making about what to do when confronted with life-and-death decisions. The problem is that, many times, physicians and other health care workers are uncomfortable with and unskilled in discussing these spiritual values with the patient. This is unfortunate because knowing a patient's religious and spiritual values and concerns can help physicians understand a patient's needs and provide that patient with respectful, comprehensive end-of-life care.[2] To understand the role of spirituality in end-of-life decision making, it is important to understand the meaning of spirituality.

Even though many in our society today talk about spirituality, it is a term that is not easily defined. Some would say, it is one of those words that, even though it is not easily defined, we know what it means when we hear it stated or see it in writing. Bioethicist Daniel Sulmasy, a Franciscan Brother and physician, has written extensively on this topic. Sulmasy suggests, "Spirituality is no more and no less than this: one's spirituality is a description of one's relationship with God. Ultimately, it is only God who can satisfy our deepest desires."[3] Spirituality is our relationship to what we ultimately value and with our commitment to live in a way that is consistent with what this value of love ultimately demands.[4] Who we are and the decisions we make should ultimately express what we love. Therefore, spirituality is a relationship of love.[5] Spirituality may name that ultimate love God, Buddha, or Allah, or it may be called the "Holy Other."

As Christians, we call this ultimate love *God*. Christian spirituality presupposes a commitment to live our lives in relation with God, revealed in Jesus Christ, as the source and end of all love, the One in whom all things have meaning and worth. Spirituality is the experience of God's transcendent love, God's overwhelming and universal concern for every person.[6] This relationship of love means that we accept God's love and become dependent on God. God loves us and expects a response from us, a response of love toward ourselves, others, the world, and ultimately, God. Spirituality is interpersonal and complex. "Spirituality takes time to develop. It waxes and wanes. It can grow warm, it can grow cold. It is a relationship that is sometimes in need of healing and forgiveness. It requires commitment despite day in and day out drudgery. It needs time alone for intimate sharing. It needs attention. It needs work."[7]

Ultimately, spirituality is about surrender to the "Voice" that calls you. It requires trust, opening oneself to the Other, allowing oneself to be loved, and allowing the Other to make demands on you.[8] Spiritual beliefs are thus fundamental to identity for many people. "Religious and spiritual variables have been associated with lower levels of mortality in prospective cohort studies, improved recovery from surgery, lower levels of substance abuse, coping with serious illness, immune function in HIV-infected patients, blood pressure control, and lower levels of health care utilization. Patients recognize the importance of these issues in their own lives, and many want physicians to consider these factors in their health care."[9] Physicians and other health care workers should appreciate the potentially beneficial role that religion and spirituality can play in the lives of individual persons. But more importantly, they have to realize how a person's spiritual beliefs and values can also affect their decision making.

It would be difficult to argue that religious faith and spirituality do not play an essential role in coping with illness and death for many patients and even physicians. It affects not only the quality of one's life but also the medical outcome. Virtually every human culture has prayed in one form or another during times of stress and the closing stages of life. Humans seem to be culturally coded to link prayer with health and death. "From the early dynasties of China to the aboriginal empires of the Americas, holy men in ancient societies ministered not only to the spiritually fallen but to the physically ill as well. In western civilization, the earliest hospitals were built, staffed, and maintained by religious orders of various denominations. This tradition has endured as religiously affiliated hospitals currently account for 20 percent of inpatient care in community hospitals and are registered with the Centers for Medicare and Medicaid Services."[10] "As early as 100,000 years ago, humans began to employ rituals when burying their dead, presumably to aid their well-being in the next life."[11]

It is clear that humans place a value on prayer and spirituality in regards to their health, but research studies on the effects of prayer and spirituality have been inconclusive. In 1872, Galton published a psychological analysis of the efficacy of prayer through a retrospective study of the effects of prayer on the health of clergy. He concluded that there were no benefits. Galton also cited an earlier study by an Englishman named Guy who concluded that the many prayers offered for the good health of British monarchs afforded them no increased longevity.[12] Others, however, found that spiritual well-being did have a positive impact on one's general health. This early interest in the effects of spirituality on health demonstrates that it is a legitimate subject of research, but the research has been far from conclusive.

Gartner et al., in the 1990s, found negative health consequences as a result of prayer. "They referred to several studies that found anxiety and fear of death to be higher in religious subjects and a tendency to have lower self-esteem. In other instances, studies of the efficacy of religious practice relative to health outcomes are inconclusive at best."[13] In 1988, Byrd's study on the efficacy of intercessory prayers was recognized as one of the most well-designed studies to date.

> Byrd reported that during a ten-month period spanning 1982 to 1983, 393 patients who were admitted to the coronary care unit of San Francisco General Hospital and were assigned randomly to either a control group (201 patients) or to a group of 192 patients for whom intercessory prayers would be offered. These patients, the staff, and physicians did not know who were in either group, and the patients were not contacted again after they had given informed consent to be part of the study. . . . Byrd concluded that the analysis of events after entry into the study showed the prayer group had less congestive heart failure, required less diuretic and antibiotic therapy, had fewer episodes of pneumonia, had fewer cardiac arrests, and were less frequently intubated and ventilated.[14]

Nevertheless, in a randomized, double-blind study in 1994 by Wirth and Mitchell on the effect of healing therapy utilizing intercessory prayer on insulin dosage in patients with type-1 diabetes mellitus, they found that although there was a reduction in insulin dosage over a period of two weeks in the treatment condition compared to the controlled condition, the difference was not statistically significant.[15]

Since 2000, at least ten other studies on the effects of prayer have been conducted—with mixed results. These studies have been done at distinguished research institutions, such as the Mind/Body Medical Institute in Boston, Duke University, and the University of Washington.[16] The most recent study is one by Herbert Benson et al. on the therapeutic effects of intercessory prayers in cardiac bypass patients.

> Patients at 6 hospitals in the United States were assigned to one of three groups: 604 received intercessory prayer after being informed that they may or may not receive prayer; 597 did not receive intercessory prayer also after being informed that they may or may not receive prayer; and 601 received intercessory prayer after being informed that they would receive prayer. Intercessory

prayer was done for 14 days starting the night before their Coronary Artery Bypass Grafting (CABG) procedure. The primary outcome was presence of any complication within 30 days of CABG. Secondary outcomes were any major event and mortality.[17]

Benson et al. found that intercessory prayer had no effect on complication-free recovery from CABG, but certainty of receiving intercessory prayer was associated with a higher incidence of complications.[18] Interestingly, one limitation of the study is that it said nothing about the power of personal prayer or about the prayers of family members and friends. The largest obstacle to any prayer study is the unknown amount of prayer each person receives from friends, family, and those around the world who pray daily for the sick and dying.[19] This study cost 2.4 million dollars and was supported by the John Templeton Foundation. To date, the federal government has spent more than $2.3 million on prayer research since 2000.[20]

Despite this most recent study, there is still considerable evidence that prayer, religious values, and spirituality can be associated with health benefits. Nevertheless, there remains considerable reluctance to integrate elements of prayer and spirituality into health care; instead they are kept on the fringes. There is a distinct gap between the practice of prayer and spirituality and the practice of medicine.[21] In a recent study on the effects of prayer on health, McCaffrey et al. found that one-third of adults used prayer for health concerns in 1998. However, most respondents did not discuss prayer with their physicians. The prayer was most often directed toward wellness and was used in conjunction with conventional medical care. Their conclusion was that "physicians should consider exploring their patients' spiritual practice to enhance their understanding of their patients' response to illness and health."[22]

In a 2004 study on patients' views about discussing spiritual issues with their physicians, Ellis and Campbell found that "regardless of religious background, patients' willingness to discuss spiritual health issues may depend on their sense of such key physician qualities as openness, nonjudgmental nature, respect for others' spiritual views, and attitudes toward spiritual health. Their views of how physicians should address spiritual issues may favor a direct, principle-based, patient-centered approach in the context of 'getting to know the patient' rather than more structured approaches such as using spiritual assessment tools."[23]

Spirituality, like health, should be viewed holistically, that is, as an integral part of the whole person. It colors the purpose and meaning that people find in life and the goals they seek. Spirituality defines context; it is not content. Research that treats spirituality as just another factor among determinants of human health misses the point. To bridge the gap between prayer and medical practice, research might need to be reconstructed within the horizon of a more holistic understanding of human health—an understanding that regards spirituality as context and humans as integrated, multifactorial beings living within a complex milieu.[24] Physicians need to gain more knowledge about and to change their attitude toward the relationship of prayer, spirituality, and medicine if they are going to be effective in understanding their patients and treating them with dignity and respect.

In seems clear that society as a whole places a value on prayer and spirituality despite the tendency within the medical establishment to move both of these to the sidelines. Studies have shown that individuals not only have engaged in prayer in an effort to improve their health or to overcome disease, but more than half of them would also welcome the opportunity to enlist their physicians in such prayerful endeavors. The problem is that physician perceptions and patient assertions simply do not seem synchronous. Most physicians are not well apprised of either the role of prayer and spirituality in health or the prayerful practices of patients because there is relatively little mention of either in health care or social science literature.[25]

In addition to this, most physicians see spirituality and prayer to be the duty of members of the pastoral care team. What they often fail to realize is that their pastoral care colleagues are part of the medical team caring for the patient. If the studies are correct in finding that religious and spiritual beliefs and practices are fundamental to the identity of most people, then physicians need to understand these beliefs and values especially as they pertain to end-of-life care. Physicians need to understand them because they are in a fiduciary relationship with their patients and have the responsibility to care for the needs of their patients. This relationship is one that is deeply human and encompasses the whole person.

"Healing requires a recognition of the human face of each person one sets out to heal and a communication of the message that both the healer and the healed share a bond that ties them to each other through their humanity, their morality, and the God-given spark of grace that lives in each of them."[26] This physician–patient relationship is a covenant based on mutual trust, honesty, compassion, and communication. Mutuality means that, on the one hand, patients need to let their physicians know their values and how these values influence their decision making. On the other hand, physicians need to be able to listen to their patients and accept their values that are based in religion and spirituality.

How discussions about spirituality are initiated between patient and physician can take various forms. In a study by Ellis and Campbell, "patients particularly valued physician initiation (on questions of spirituality) in cases of 'chronic illness that relates to death and dying' as opposed to less serious presentations. Conversely, one respondent observed that serious illness empowers patients to initiate discussions despite their preference for doctor initiation."[27] This study also revealed that patients felt that when physicians talk about spirituality they are acknowledging their limitations in their power to heal, which reassures the patient that they know God has the ultimate power.

Patients also expressed their concern that physicians know the difference between being an encourager versus a spiritual advisor. Understanding the appropriate boundaries gives patients the feeling of being empowered to set the agenda of spiritual discussions. Patients appreciate physician openness but disdain proselytizing. Patients also felt that physicians should know their limitations and utilize pastoral professionals when they need expertise in this area.[28] This study makes it clear that Americans draw on religious and spiritual beliefs when confronted with serious illness, especially with end-of-life issues, and that physicians have a responsibility to be knowledgeable and sensitive about spirituality. Having this technical competence is an integral part of the physician–patient relationship.

In a recent cross-sectional survey of 2,000 practicing U.S. clinicians in which 63 percent responded, 56 percent of clinicians believed that religion and spirituality had much or very much influence on health, but only 6 percent believed that religion and spirituality often changed "hard" medical outcomes. In contrast, most clinicians believed that religion and spirituality often helps patients cope (76 percent), puts patients in a positive frame of mind (75 percent), and provides emotional and practical support via the religious community (55 percent).[29] The major problem is that many physicians lack the skills and even feel uncomfortable discussing spiritual and religious concerns with patients.[30]

Lo et al. give some practical suggestions about how to respond when patients and family members raise spiritual and religious concerns:

> First, some patients may explicitly base decisions about life-sustaining interventions on their spiritual or religious beliefs. Physicians need to explore those beliefs to help patients think through

their preferences regarding specific interventions. Second, other patients may not bring up spiritual or religious concerns but are troubled by them. Physicians should identify such concerns and listen to them empathetically, without trying to alleviate the patient's spiritual suffering or offering premature reassurance. Third, some patients or families may have religious reasons for insisting on life-sustaining interventions that physicians advise against. The physician should listen and try to understand the patient's viewpoint. Listening respectfully does not require the physician to agree with the patient or misrepresent his or her own views. Patients and families who feel that the physician understands them and cares about them may be more willing to consider the physician's views on prognosis and treatment.[31]

When dealing with patients who are trying to make a decision about whether to initiate life-sustaining interventions, Lo et al. believe the following can be used to elicit the patient's concerns:

1. Use open-ended questions. Examples: Does your trust in God lead you to think about cardiopulmonary resuscitation in a particular way? Do you have any thoughts about why this is happening?

2. Ask the patient to say more. Examples: Tell me more about that. Can you tell me how you think your mother is suffering?

3. Acknowledge and normalize the patient's concerns. Example: Many patients ask the same type of questions.

4. Use empathic comments. Examples: I imagine I would feel pretty puzzled to not know. That sounds like a painful situation.

5. Ask about the patient's emotions. Examples: How do you feel about moving toward palliative care? How has it been for you with your wife in the intensive care unit for so long?[32]

There are also pitfalls when a physician is having a discussion with a patient about spiritual and religious issues near the end of life. The following should be avoided:

1. Trying to solve the patient's problems or resolve unanswerable questions.
2. Going beyond the physician's expertise and role, or imposing the physician's religious beliefs on the patient. Providing premature reassurance.[33]

Understanding the religious and spiritual beliefs of a patient can help physicians understand certain treatment decisions made by patients and can also give physicians the ability to provide the necessary support for patients and their families. The following are guidelines for physicians when discussing spiritual and religious issues with patients and families near the end of life:

1. Clarify the patient's concerns, beliefs, values, and needs, and follow hints about spiritual and religious issues.
2. Make a connection with the patient by listening carefully, acknowledging the patient's concerns, exploring emotions, and using wish statements.
3. Identify common goals for care and reach agreement on clinical decisions.
4. Mobilize sources of support for the patient and the family.[34]

These are guidelines that can help physicians better understand their patients—especially their spiritual and religious concerns as they are confronted with the end-of-life decisions. By listening and responding to these concerns, physicians may also help their patients find comfort and closure as they near the end of life.[35]

After examining the literature and listening to patients and physicians in acute-care facilities as they confront terminal illnesses together, it is clear that there is a connection between spirituality and health. The beneficial effects of religion and spirituality are neither universal nor reproducible, however, and are complicated by numerous confounding factors.[36] Despite all the studies and recent literature in medical journals on this topic, there is still a silence concerning how physicians and other health care professionals perceive spirituality in terms of health benefits. Until this silence is broken, our goal of helping patients die with dignity and respect will remain illusive.

When patients make end-of-life decisions, they do so based on their long-held values that are, most often, rooted in their religious and spiritual beliefs. Understanding a patient's religious values and initiating a conversation with the patient about the options available can help bridge the gap that is often present when a patient has been informed that further treatments are no longer beneficial and hospice or palliative care is recommended. But just understanding a patient's spiritual values is not enough. Physicians and health care professionals must also walk with patients and be present to patients as they face the inevitability of death. This is important because there exists a void between the time a terminally ill patient is informed that further medical treatment is useless and the initiation of palliative or hospice care.

During this period of time the potential exists for a terminally ill patient to be confronted with two distinct options. First, the patient can be overwhelmed by the fear of suffering and death, which can result in feelings of abandonment and despair. Second, the patient can, with the support of loved ones and understanding health care professionals, accept the inevitability of suffering and death and grow in his or her dependence upon others and God. This time of transition also exists for family members and friends of the terminally ill patient and even for health care professionals. They too are confronted with two distinct options. They can avoid the inevitable by isolating the patient in the hospital, under the guise of what is best for the patient, which can often lead to feelings of guilt and remorse after the death of the patient. Or, they can support the terminally ill patient by their loving presence, which allows family members and friends—and, to a certain extent, health care professionals—to face their deepest fears and to embrace death as part of the normal cycle of life.

For the patient as well as for family and health care professionals, this period of transition is crucial because, within this time frame, the bond of relationship between them is transformed. This transformation can become either the basis for alienation and despair, or the essence of acceptance and hope. Unless the disparity between these two options is clearly understood, there is little hope that the patient will die with dignity and respect. Understanding these two options from within a spiritual framework of values and beliefs can help the patient find not only comfort but even peace of mind as the inevitability of death approaches. For this to happen, we need to understand these two options that confront the patient.

FEAR OF ABANDONMENT

Suffering and death are facts of life, yet most aspects of American culture foster denial of the ultimate reality. Many Americans don't think about death, talk about death, or even want to see it. We have become a "death-denying" society. As a result, the American culture has created a "conspiracy of silence" when confronted with suffering and death. Those who are critically ill and are suspected of being terminally ill tend to be separated from the healthy in society—including their family and friends. They are sent off to hospitals, with all good intentions, where they enter the strange and impersonal world of medical care. These patients are barraged with innumerable medical tests and procedures, they are attached to the latest in medical technology, and for all intents and purposes, appear to be getting the best medical care insurance can provide. But in reality, they are beginning a long process that for many can result in feeling dehumanized.

Many become just another patient, in a particular room, with a specific disease. Who they are—what they have done, and where they come from—becomes lost in the world of clinical medicine. In the beginning, family and friends visit frequently and physicians are positive and upbeat, but gradually, these visits become less frequent and attitudes become less positive when the diagnosis reveals that the patient is terminal and the prognosis gives the patient only a matter of months to live. For many families and even physicians, the first reaction is to give the loved one or patient false hope. The "conspiracy of silence" takes on a new dynamism. Variations of chemotherapy, radiation therapy, experimental medications, and surgeries are attempted, but, in the end, all prove to be nonbeneficial. Instead of facing the inevitability of death through honest dialogue, family members and physicians continue the "conspiracy of silence" until they reach the point when the patient has to be told that further medical treatment is useless. It is then that loved ones and even physicians can begin to experience feelings of distance and detachment and the patient is confronted with feelings of abandonment and despair. The terminal patient begins to learn that suffering not only alienates one from others but it can also alienate one from oneself.

Instead of being sensitive to the needs of the terminally ill to talk about their condition and the time they may have left, family, friends, and even physicians often distance themselves from the issue at hand and the person in particular. Avoidance and artificiality become the norm. At a time when a frank and loving conversation about death and dying would benefit all concerned, many today revert to denial.

This avoidance of the inevitable is having a profound impact on our culture. In the past, the elderly and the terminally ill died at home comforted by family and friends. Their physicians were oftentimes even present at the bedside when they died. Today, many elderly and terminally ill patients end their earthly existence alone in a hospital feeling useless and abandoned. The distance and silence that results from this insensitivity leads many terminally ill patients to dwell upon the negative aspects of life. They fear becoming a financial and emotional burden to family and society. They begin to realize that their many dreams and aspirations will never be realized, thus their failures and disappointments become magnified. They begin to question the basic religious and spiritual values that dominated their lives, which now seem to offer little satisfaction. Finally, society has shown them firsthand how their impending loss of autonomy can lead to feelings of vulnerability, which only increases their sense of fear. They have witnessed the fear of isolation, degradation, and humiliation, which they know can lead to the possibility of exploitation, manipulation, and abuse. It is this sense of fear and feelings of abandonment and loneliness that can lead many terminally ill patients to despair. And, it is this sense of despair that is the driving force behind the current debate on the issue of "dying well," that is, with "dignity and respect." As a result, physician-assisted suicide is on the horizon, and it is becoming a haunting reality for many who are terminally ill.

It need not be such a haunting reality. There is a viable option that can assist both patient and loved ones. It is an option that truly allows a person to die with dignity and respect. That option is palliative and hospice care, which allows a patient to die comfortably and at peace, surrounded by loved ones with dignity and respect. But for this option to become a reality, family members, friends, and even physicians must commit themselves to be present to the terminally ill patient, and the terminally ill patient must allow himself or herself to become dependent on them as well.

THE HOPE OF ACCEPTANCE THROUGH DEPENDENCE ON OTHERS AND GOD

With the initiation of palliative care and the emergence of hospice care, many terminally ill patients, family members, and physicians have been given the opportunity to face suffering and death together with a new sense of honesty and dignity. Suffering and death no longer need to be feared and avoided, but can be faced with courage and acceptance. The Christian tradition has always argued that pain and suffering have a special place in God's saving plan. Without glorifying suffering, the Christian tradition has viewed suffering and even death within a larger perspective, that of the redemptive process. By suffering, Christians can participate in the paschal mystery. Ethicist Richard McCormick argues that "suffering is not mere pain and confusion, dying is not merely an end. These must be viewed, even if mysteriously, in terms of a larger process: as occasions for a growing self-opening after Christ's example, as various participations in the paschal mystery."[37] For the Christian, pain and suffering must be seen as something more than that which is to be avoided.

Christians view life within the context of the Christian mysteries. McCormick believes, "just as Christ suffered and died for us to enter his glory, so we who are 'in the Lord,' who are inserted into the redemptive mystery, must expect that our growth 'to deeper life' will share the characteristics of God's engendering deed in Christ."[38] Grave illness is to be seen as an intensifying conformity to Christ. As the human body weakens and is devastated by disease and illness, the strength of Jesus Christ is shared by those who have been baptized into his death and resurrection. This conviction reinforces the view that human persons are completely dependent upon God's love.

Christ manifested his supreme dignity by doing God's will—"Not my will, but thine be done" (Luke 22:42). Christians are called to that same dependence on God's love that Christ showed on the Cross. This dependence on God manifests itself in our human dependence upon others. Therefore, suffering should lead not only to dependence on God, but to dependence on others. When a person is experiencing pain and suffering, that person needs the help and presence of others. Only through dependence on others and God can one become truly independent.

To understand the full implications of being dependent on others and God, ethicist Drew Christiansen, S.J., developed a "theology of dependence." Christiansen argues that being dependent on others is an inescapable part of being human. For most of our lives, however, we ignore this sense of dependence that binds us to one another. We strive to be self-sufficient, but we will never reach our goal. As finite creatures, we only deceive ourselves by thinking we are in control and that we do not need to rely upon others—and thus to rely on God. Christiansen believes that our fear of dependence is misplaced if it is divorced from the Christian approach to it. "Our natural desire is to hold on as long as possible, to maintain our independence, to go it alone. From a faith stance, however, it is possible to let go, to accept support from others, and to find fulfillment in a community of care."[39]

Outside of faith, we fear that dependence threatens us with subjugation. But for the Christian, the promise hidden in dependence is a fuller communion with the Source of Life.[40] In the mystery of suffering "we are invited to let go of certainties and trust that the mystery in which we have our being—God—is benevolent toward us."[41] Letting go of our control and overcoming our fear of dependence can only be accomplished if God is made present to the terminally ill patient through the love and presence of others.

Being present to another must occur in both words and actions. It is not enough to tell a terminally ill patient to have courage because Christ is suffering with him or her. We must be Christ for that person by our loving presence. Family members, friends, and health care professionals must become "silent signs" of God's love and presence by entering into the suffering of the terminally ill patient—not peripherally, but in an intimate and loving way. Such presence allows the terminally ill patient to realize that he or she is not alone. God is present in the presence of others. Through this loving presence of others, the terminally ill patient finds hope which challenges him or her to keep looking and listening because it now makes sense to hope.

Why would God abandon me at such an important moment? God did not abandon Job. Instead, God called Job to a deeper personal relationship with God through self-surrender. The terminally ill patient is also being called to self-surrender, that is, to place one's suffering before God, and to trust in God's unconditional love. This self-surrender can only be accomplished with the love and commitment of family, friends, and health care professionals. To foster this sense of loving presence and to bridge the transition that exists between termination of medical treatment and the beginning of palliative or hospice care, there is a need for a formal ritual that will strengthen the bond of Christian commitment between the patient and his or her family and physicians. The ritual proposed is one called the "Rite of Commitment to the Terminally Ill." This ritual was designed to help not only the patient, but also the family members and health care professionals, to understand the importance of a person's spiritual values and the responsibility we have toward one another as humans and as Christians.

THE RITE OF CHRISTIAN COMMITMENT TO THE TERMINALLY ILL

During times of crisis and periods of transition, a ritual can play a significant role in the emergence and resolution of such phases. A ritual can be understood as a social, symbolic process which has the potential for communicating, creating, criticizing, and even transforming meaning. It is a dynamic system of symbols, a process constituted by symbols and their significations. Ritual symbols can be any object, activity, relationship, word, gesture, or spacial arrangement which serves as a unit in the ritual process. The major benefit of a ritual is that new relationships may be formed and previous relationships among participants may be strengthened.[42]

The purpose of this particular ritual is for those who minister to the sick and dying to bring together the terminally ill person with family, friends, and health care professionals at this moment of transition, so that the bond of relationship between them can be strengthened in the presence of God and one another. As a ritual symbol, family members, friends, and health care professionals will commit themselves in both word and action to be present to the terminally ill patient throughout the remainder of his or her illness and when possible, the patient accepts their commitment. Just as Christ showed great concern for the bodily and spiritual welfare of the sick and dying by his presence to them, so family members, friends, and health care professionals, as fellow humans (and sometimes as Christians), will commit themselves in the "Rite of Christian Commitment to the Terminally Ill" to do the same. The following is an outline of the "Rite of Christian Commitment to the Terminally Ill":

I. Introductory Rites:

A. Greeting
P. The peace of the Lord be with you always.
R. And also with you.

B. Instruction:
My dear brothers and sisters, the Lord Jesus, who went about doing good works and healing sickness and infirmity of every kind, commanded his disciples to lovingly care for the sick and dying, to pray for them, and to lay hands on them. In this celebration, we shall entrust our sick brothers and sisters to the care of the Lord, asking that he will enable them to bear their pain and suffering in the knowledge that, if they accept their share in the pain of his passion, they will also share in its power to give comfort and strength. We ask this through Christ our Lord. Amen.[43]

II. Liturgy of the Word
A. Suggested Readings:

Hebrew Scripture
1. Psalm 23
2. Psalm 71
3. Job 7: 1–4, 6–11
4. Job 7: 12–21
5. Job 19: 23–27
6. Isaiah 35: 1–10
7. Isaiah 52: 13–53:12
8. Isaiah 61: 1–3
9. Wisdom 9: 1, 9–18

New Testament
1. 2 Corinthians 1: 3–7
2. Romans 8: 31b–35, 37–39
3. Romans 8: 18–27
4. Colossians 1:22–29
5. Matthew 5: 1–12
6. Matthew 11: 28–30
7. Luke 12: 22–32
8. John 6: 35–40
9. John 6: 53–58

III. Prayers of Christian Commitment
(The pastoral care member will begin by introducing the individual prayers of Christian commitment with a short prayer calling upon God to give comfort and care to the person who is ill. Then, each person present will extemporaneously present a prayer for the person who is ill stating his/her intention to be present to the person who is ill throughout the remainder of their illness. The patient, if possible, will then state his/her intention to allow family, friends, and health care professionals to be present to him/her.)

Introduction:
Jesus came as healer of body and of spirit in order to cure all our ills. He chose to be like us in all things, in order to assure us of his compassion. He bore our weakness and carried our sorrows. He felt compassion for the crowd, and went about doing good and healing the sick. With trust, let us pray to Jesus that he will comfort (N.) with his grace and that he will fill (N.) with new hope and strength.

Family, Friends, and Health Care Professionals:

I pray that Christ will comfort you as you follow him on the path he has set before you. As your (family member /

friend / health care professional), I promise to walk with you on your journey. I promise I will be present to you in both word and action. Just as Jesus felt compassion for the crowd, and went about doing good by caring for them, I promise that I will watch over you, that I will be there when you need me, and that I will show you the love of Christ by my very presence. (N.), in the presence of God and all present, I commit myself to you with the love of Jesus Christ.

Patient:
I accept your commitment to walk with me as I face my illness in the days ahead. I thank God for your love and your presence to me and acknowledge how blessed I am to have you all in my life.

IV. Prayer of Blessing
(All present will extend their hands over the person who is ill and pray the following prayer. At the conclusion of the prayer, each person will trace the sign of the cross on the forehead of the person who is ill.)

Lord, our God, you sent your only begotten Son into the world to bear our infirmities and to endure our sufferings. Look with compassion upon your servant (N.). Give (him/her) strength in body, courage in spirit, and patience in pain. Support (N.) with your grace, comfort (him/her) with your protection, and give (him/her) the strength to fight against all evil. Since you have given (N.) a share in your own passion, help (him/her) to find hope and consolation in suffering, for you are Lord for ever and ever. Amen.

All: Our Father, who art in heaven . . .

V. Concluding Rite:
God of mercy, look kindly on your servant (N.), who has grown weak under the burden of illness. Strengthen (him/her) by your grace and help (him/her) to remain close

to you in prayer. Fill (him/her) with the strength of your
Holy Spirit. Keep (him/her) strong in faith and serene in
hope, so that (he/she) may give us all an example of patience, and joyfully witness to the power of your love.
Lord, we ask you to soothe the hearts of the family members and friends of (N.) gathered here today. In your loving
kindness, enlighten their faith, give hope to their hearts,
and peace to their lives. We ask this through Christ our
Lord. Amen.

Dismissal:
Go in the peace of Christ to serve him in the sick and in all who
need your love.[44]

This ritual may not be applicable for all patients who are terminally
ill because of their specific faith beliefs. However, it can be modified to
meet the needs of various other faiths. The main point is that all present—
patient, family members, friends, and health care professionals—commit
themselves to be present to the patient during the illness and promise that
they will walk with the patient to the conclusion. Such a process has the
power not only to strengthen relationships but to transform them for the
good of all.

CONCLUSION

Clinical medicine and religious and spiritual values and beliefs are
from two distinct worlds and can represent two very different subcultures
in our society. Medicine aspires to be objective and scientific; spirituality
and religious beliefs are subjective and faith-oriented. Health care professionals are taught to keep a professional distance; believers seek communion with the community and the world. Tension between these two ways
of interpreting experience comes to the surface when confronting the ultimate decisions at the end of life.[45] The gap between spirituality and medical
practice can be bridged if there is an open, honest dialogue between patients, family members, and health care professionals. Taking the time to
understand the values and beliefs of a patient, helping patients think
through their values and beliefs as they pertain to medical interventions,
listening empathetically and respectfully to patients as they explain their
viewpoints, and having a holistic understanding of human health can help
alleviate many tensions that confront people at the end of life.

Physicians can no longer remain silent when issues of spirituality and prayer surface nor can they fear exploring their patients' spiritual practices. Studies have shown that prayer and spirituality may improve quality of life—enhancing a person's subjective well-being by providing coping strategies, stress relief, and social support.[46] Exploring a patient's spiritual and religious values and beliefs will only enhance a physician's understanding of that patient's response to illness and health. The debate within the medical profession about the appropriate place of spirituality in patient care will continue. Many will continue to require substantive evidence that there are objective health outcomes. Others will lower their defenses and begin to dialogue with their patients so that when decisions are made at the end of life, they will understand the basis of their decision making and will be empathetic toward the ways spirituality allows patients to cope with suffering and death. When this dialogue occurs, then the true meaning of spirituality that is grounded in the love of God and others will transform the experience of dying and will allow patients to die with real dignity and respect.

EIGHT:
CONCLUSION

An intense preoccupation with the preservation of physical life, however, seems sometimes to be based on an assumption that death is unnatural, or that its delay, even briefly, through medical and technical means is always a triumph of human achievement over the limitations of nature. It is as if death is in every case an evil, a kind of demonic power to be overcome by the forces of life, propped up by elaborate medical technologies. Dramatic interventions portrayed in the media become living "westerns." The powers of death are the bad guys, to be vanquished by the good guys, dressed in white coats rather than white hats. Every delay of death is a victory by the forces of good. Or, to change the analogy, the development and use of costly and dramatic end-stage therapies are seen as the "arms" to be used in a "crusade," a war fought over "holy places" because they were occupied by an alien, and therefore an enemy, power. A "crusading mentality" comes into being; almost any means is justified when it will delay the enemy, death.[1]

To die with dignity and respect is not an easy task, because dying is never dignified. There is a fear of the unknown, a fear of dying alone, a fear of pain and indignity, and a fear of being a burden to others. But death is not the enemy. The enemies are unnecessary suffering, avoidance, and abandonment.

As caregivers, our goal is to give those who are dying, by our very presence and care, a reason to hope. As Christians, we are called to be Christ—in both word and action—for those who are suffering. "We are to do for others what Jesus did: comfort others by inspiring in them hope and confidence in life. As God's ongoing, creative acting in the world and the love of Christ make it possible for us to continue to live despite the chaos of illness, so too our work in the world must also give hope to those for whom we care."[2] Illness, especially terminal illness, can remove those individuals from the community. The terminally ill patient is often separated from the healthy in society including their family and friends. It is said we do this so that the patient can receive the best in medical treatment and care, but in reality, often it is done to protect us—family and friends.

The patient is moved from the comfort of his or her home, sent to the hospital, with all good intentions, where he or she enters the unfamiliar and impersonal world of medical care. The patient is barraged with numerous tests and procedures, attached to the latest in medical technology, and for all intents and purposes appears to be getting the best medical care in the world. However, in reality, it is the beginning of a long process of isolation and dehumanization. The patient becomes a nameless subject in a particular room with a specific disease. Who she is, what he has accomplished, where she comes from—all seem to be lost in the world of clinical medicine. With the diagnosis of a terminal illness, the "conspiracy of silence" becomes a reality.

Instead of talking about the emotions the patient is feeling, the desires of what he or she wants to accomplish before death, or any fears and anxieties, a new dynamism of "false hope" comes to the surface. Rather than initiating an honest dialogue with the patient about hospice and palliative care, new alternatives are given—additional chemotherapy and radiation, or an experimental drug protocol, or one more surgery. This is when the patient is confronted by the forces of good and evil—death with dignity or life at any cost.

On the one hand, the patient can play into the "conspiracy of silence" and accept further aggressive treatment that will in the end prove to be nonbeneficial. Or, on the other hand, an open, honest discussion can begin with the patient, family, and physician about the reality of the terminal illness, accepting the inevitable that cannot be changed, and letting go of our control on a situation that is in reality uncontrollable. It is at this point that the patient who has been removed from the community because of illness can be welcomed back into the community because his or her health, in a broad sense, has been restored. The patient understands the reality of the situation and accepts the inevitable. This is the beginning of hope, a hope that can rise from the ashes like the ancient phoenix, and avoid the opposite of hope, which is despair. For this hope to become a reality, it needs to be nourished, and everyone has a role to play.

Family and friends must become the "bearers of hope," by committing themselves to walk with their loved one as they walk toward death. To quote the prophet Isaiah, "No need to recall the past, no need to think about what was done before. See, I am doing a new deed, even now it comes to light; can you not see it?" (Isaiah 43: 18–19). As bearers of hope, we know that the new can only come about by the collapse of the old. The patient's life is changed, not ended. Being present to the patient in word and action will encourage the patient to face each day with a spirit of hope. This loving presence also lets the patient know that he is important and valued— that she is not alone and will not be alone. The patient realizes that he or she is part of a loving community that is hope-filled.

This presence by family and friends is also very practical. As the patient grows weaker, simple daily tasks that most of us take for granted become more complex and finally impossible to do. This can be a crushing blow to hope unless there is someone there to say, "It is ok to let go, to become dependent on me, because I am here for you." The simplest loss of function is a constant reminder of the inevitability of death. This is when our presence becomes a sign of hope for the patient. We now hope for them until they can hope for themselves again. The temptation for many is to avoid the terminal patient and run as far and fast as possible from them. The focus of this fear is not on the loved one who is suffering and dying from a terminal illness but on our own fear of mortality. Seeing a mother, father, brother, sister, or friend lying in a bed and dying stirs in us the reality that we too are going to die and that we have no real control over the situation. Being present to the patient enables us to face our fears and to look them straight in the eye. Then and only then will they become less fearful. Fear drives us to avoid the situation; hope allows us to face it head-on.

Physicians and other health care professionals are also integral to the process of hope. Many health care professionals have a tendency, when confronted with a terminal patient, to hide behind their clinical skills and professional demeanor. They have been trained not to get too involved with their patients for fear that they will lose their objectivity. So they hide behind a clinical diagnosis and prognosis and begin to treat symptoms. They also hide behind the professional role of the physician. These facades, however, become far too transparent to both patients and family members.

A false sense of bravado and professionalism does not play well if one is facing the inevitability of death. What is called for in these situations is a humanness that is grounded in honesty and compassion. Physicians, as human persons and as medical professionals, are called to seek the truth. Yes, it might be easier to sugarcoat the inevitable terminal prognosis by offering the false hope of an additional round of chemotherapy or an experimental drug protocol, but in reality, deceiving and exaggerating do not help the patient, the family, or even the physician. Delivering bad news or discussing other end-of-life issues is never easy. It is a skill that has to be learned. The basis of such a skill is being honest with the patient and being there for the patient until the very end.

Physicians must also be able to acknowledge and process their own feelings which arise when caring for a dying patient. Often, physicians fail to realize that they are not alone in caring for a dying patient. They work as a team with nurses, social workers, pastoral care chaplains, and their fellow physicians.[3] Physicians and health care professionals need to be present to the patient, but it is equally important for the health care team to be present also to one another, in order to give support, encouragement, and hope. As health care professionals, physicians are expected to have expertise in clinical medicine, but they are also called to be compassionate.

Sulmasy gives three levels on which physicians can engage the suffering of a patient in a compassionate way. "First, the compassionate clinician is the one who objectively recognizes the suffering of the patient, giving it a name and understanding its natural history. Second, the compassionate clinician is the one who subjectively responds to this suffering with feelings of genuine empathy for the patient, striving to understand the situation of the patient as experienced by the patient. Third, the compassionate clinician is the one who is moved to concrete healing actions—words and deeds."[4] Compassionate physicians are called to heal and care for the whole person. When a physician can no longer heal, he or she can still care for the patient.

Both physicians and family members are called to be present to a patient who is terminally ill in both word and action. Being present will not only help the patient as he or she nears the end of life, it will also give family members and physicians the abilities to help the next person they encounter who is dying. Each time we walk with a person who is dying, we learn more about the process of dying and death. As a professor of medical ethics, I tell my students that I consider myself a student of dying and death. Being both a Catholic priest and a bioethicist, I have the privilege of walking with many people as they face the end of life. Most of my teachers of dying and death have been children since my area of specialty is neonatology and pediatrics. Each child I have walked with who has died has better prepared me to deal with the next child and his or her family undergoing the dying process.

Being present for my father's death due to Alzheimer's disease better prepared me to walk with my mother as she died from a prolonged illness. Together with my sister, we had the privilege to be present when each of them—our father and our mother—died. We had cared for them together during their illnesses, and at the end we stood by each of them, holding their hands as they slipped away peacefully. This was an experience of dying with dignity and respect. Walking with loved ones as they experience intense suffering and face the inevitability of death is the simplest and most difficult thing we can do. It is simple because all one has to do is be present and be there. It is difficult because our natural instinct is to run for our lives.

Our powerlessness can be excruciating at such times.[5] But the reality of the experience is that it will only make us stronger and will allow us to face the next experience with a loved one or a patient with even more compassion and greater hope. We are called as humans to be individuals in a community. As such, each of us has the responsibility to help our fellow brothers and sisters, to be present to them, and to never abandon them, especially as they near the end of life. Each of us has the ability to foster hope in another. When there is no longer hope for a cure, there is still hope for a good quality of life. As humans, we have the responsibility to be present throughout the end-of-life caring process.

There will be occasions when patients are alone. Family members and friends are not present and physicians are aloof and treating the disease instead of the whole person. To assure patients that they are empowered to participate in their treatment decisions, three safeguards have been put in place. The problem is that many people are unaware of these safeguards. First, patients have the right to name a durable power of attorney for health care who, after discussions with the patient, understands the patient's values and knows what the patient would want in the event that he or she becomes incompetent. Knowing there is someone there who will make a substituted judgment for you can be very reassuring. Second, patients also have the ability to write a living will or advance directive. These documents state what the patient would want in the event that the patient is incompetent and is either permanently unconscious or has an end-stage condition. They allow the patient to participate in treatment decisions even after the patient has become incompetent. They also lessen the possibility of feelings of guilt and even friction among family members under difficult situations, and they give direction to physicians about what is in the best interest of the patient.

In addition to respecting the patient's right of autonomy regarding medical treatments, these documents will also help to ensure the responsible use of medical resources. Terminal illness imposes substantial burdens—economic and otherwise—on patients, caregivers, and society as a whole.[6] Many of the treatments that patients receive at the end of life are unnecessary, medically futile, and extremely expensive. There are approximately 47 million people in the United States without health care. Spending money on medically futile treatments is not only nonbeneficial for the patient but is an injustice for society as a whole.

Third, there may be instances when the patients and family members get into confrontations with the physician about end-of-life treatments. Most of these scenarios are due to a lack of communication or a miscommunication that ends up putting all parties into an adversarial situation. One example is when a patient is requesting aggressive medical treatment and the physician believes it is futile treatment but the patient is threatening legal action because his or her right of autonomy is being violated. This is a situation when an ethics consultation might be beneficial.

After hospice, the second-best-kept secret in a hospital is the presence of an ethics committee. An institutional ethics committee is a multidisciplinary group comprising about 15 to 20 members, whose function is threefold: to educate regarding biomedical issues, to develop and review institutional policies, and to serve in an advisory capacity in bioethical disputes. As an advisory group, the ethics committee should consider and assist in resolving unusual, complicated ethical problems involving issues that affect care and treatment of patients within the health care institution. "Recommendations of the ethics committee should impose no obligation for acceptance on the part of the institution, its governing board, medical staff, attending physician, or other persons. However, it should be expected that the recommendations of a dedicated ethics committee will receive serious consideration by decision makers."[7] Access to ethics committees is open to all involved in patient-care decisions including the patient and the patient's family. This mechanism for resolving disputes should be available in every hospital so that the rights of patients, physicians, and society as a whole are protected. Patients and family members who find themselves in an adversarial situation with their attending physician over a medical-ethical dilemma should be aware of the existence of the hospital ethics committee and should be helped to access a consultation.

As a society that claims to be at the forefront of modern medicine, our focus continues to be one that in practice is a "fix-it" mentality. With daily advances in medicine and technology, treatment options for patients seem unlimited. The curative care approach to medicine is still the dominant approach in western medicine. But with the advent of hospice care and a movement among many in the medical profession to advocate for transitioning to a palliative care approach, patients are beginning to realize that they do have more options when faced with a terminal disease.[8]

This new approach is not only good for patients, but also for physicians and society as a whole. Patients are being given an honest and complete evaluation of their condition so that they have all the facts to make an informed decision between aggressive treatment and palliative care. Physicians are learning to accept the finitude of medicinal treatments but at the same time the fullness of medical care. And society is being benefited because the palliative care approach is ensuring a responsible stewardship of medical resources which will benefit all in society. When patients are given all the options open to them at the end of life, including hospice and palliative care, adequate pain assessment and management, and spiritual and social support for themselves and their family, then they will experience full quality-of-life care and be able to die with dignity and respect.

Death is not the enemy. "The real enemies are disease, discomfort, disability, fear, and anxiety. Sensitive, perceptive physicians attempt to guide their patients, those who are relatively healthy as well as those who are seriously handicapped and ill, to a perspective in which preservation of life is not their God."[9] As humans, we are born, we live, and then we die. Death is part of the natural cycle of life. For Christians, death is a transition; life as we know it has changed but has not ended. Hope allows us to celebrate both life and death. It is our duty as persons, whether we are family members, friends, or health care professionals, to understand life and death within the context of hope so that we can help our loved ones to die with dignity and respect. There is no greater gift we can give to a person than our presence during this last segment of the journey of life.

1

Notes

Introduction

[1] Steinhauser et al., "In Search of a Good Death," 829.
[2] Ibid.
[3] Sheehan, "A Great Comfort."
[4] Steinhauser et al., 829.
[5] Ibid., 827.
[6] Sheehan, "On Dying Well."
[7] Kübler-Ross, *On Death and Dying.*
[8] Steinhauser et al., 826–828.
[9] For a more detailed evaluation of SPIKES, see Baile et al. "SPIKES—A Six-Step Protocol for Delivering Bad News: Application to the Patient with Cancer."
[10] Ibid., 6–10.

One: Definition of Death, Consciousness, and Persistent Vegetative State

[1] Lazar et al., "Bioethics for Clinicians: 24. Brain Death," 833. See also Wertheimer, Jouvet, and Descotes, "A Propos du Diagnostic de la Mort du Système Nerveux les Comas avec Arrêt Respiratoire Traités par Respiration Artificielle."
[2] Crippen, "Brain Failure and Brain Death: Introduction."
[3] Doig and Burgess, "Brain Death: Resolving Inconsistencies in the Ethical Declaration of Death." See also, Powner, Ackerman, and Grenvik, "Medical Diagnosis of Death in Adults: Historical Contributions to Current Controversies."
[4] Rubenstein, Cohen, and Jackson, "The Definition of Death and the Ethics of Organ Procurement from the Deceased," 7.
[5] Ibid., 2.
[6] Ibid., 7.
[7] Ad Hoc Committee of the Harvard Medical School to Examine the Definition of Brain Death, "A Definition of Irreversible Coma."
[8] Ibid.
[9] Rubenstein, Cohen, and Jackson, "The Definition of Death," 8.
[10] Those who advocate for a "higher-brain-oriented criteria" maintain that permanent cessation of all mental functions of the human person should be equated

with death. This has the potential of classifying a larger class of patients as dead.

[11] Halevy and Brody, "Brain Death: Reconciling Definitions, Criteria, and Tests."

[12] President's Commission for the Study of Ethical Problems in Medicine and Biomedical and Behavioral Research, "Defining Death: A Report on the Medical, Legal and Ethical Issues in the Determination of Death."

[13] Medical Consultants on the Diagnosis of Death to the President's Commission for the Study of Ethical Problems in Medicine and Biomedical and Behavioral Research, "Guidelines for the Determination of Death."

[14] Uniform Definition of Death Act. 12 Uniform Laws Annotated 320 (1990 Supp). See also note 13 above.

[15] Halevy and Brody, "Brain Death," 520.

[16] Freer, "Brain Death."

[17] Lazar et al., "Bioethics for Clinicians: 24. Brain Death," 834.

[18] Freer, "Brain Death," 1.

[19] "Brain Death—Well Settled Yet Still Unresolved."

[20] Morioka, "Reconsidering Brain Death: A Lesson from Japan's Fifteen Years Experience," 41–42. See also, Olick, "Brain Death, Religious Freedom, and Public Policy," 285.

[21] Freer, "Brain Death," 1.

[22] Lazar et al., "Bioethics for Clinicians: 24. Brain Death," 834.

[23] Multi-Society Task Force on PVS, "Medical Aspects of the Persistent Vegetative State—First of Two Parts."

[24] Jennett and Plum, "Persistent Vegetative State after Brain Damage: A Syndrome in Search of a Name."

[25] Quality Standards Subcommittee of the American Academy of Neurology, "Practice Parameters: Assessment and Management of Patients in a Persistent Vegetative State."

[26] Ibid.; Multi-Society Task Force on PVS, "Medical Aspects of the Persistent Vegetative State—First of Two Parts," 1499; and Working Group of the Royal College of Physicians, "The Permanent Vegetative State."

[27] Quality Standards Subcommittee of the American Academy of Neurology, "Practice Parameters," 1016–1017.

[28] *Acute traumatic and nontraumatic brain injury*: PVS usually evolves within one month of injury from a state of eyes-closed coma to a state of wakefulness without awareness with sleep–wake cycles and preserved brainstem functions.

Degenerative and metabolic disorders of the brain: Many degenerative and metabolic nervous-system disorders in adults and children inevitably progress toward an irreversible vegetative state. Patients who are severely impaired but retain some degree of awareness may lapse briefly into a vegetative state from the effects of medication, infection, superimposed illnesses, or decreased fluid and nutritional intake. Such temporary encephalopathy must be corrected before establishing that the patient is in PVS. If the vegetative state persists for several months, recovery of consciousness is unlikely.

Severe developmental malformations of the nervous system: The developmental vegetative state is a form of PVS that affects some infants and children with severe congenital malformations of the nervous system. These children do not acquire awareness of the self or the environment. This diagnosis can be made at birth only with infants with anencephaly. For children with other severe malformations who appear vegetative at birth, observation for three to six months is recommended to determine whether these infants acquire awareness. The majority of such infants who are vegetative at birth remain vegetative; those who acquire awareness usually recover only to a severe disability. See Quality Standards Subcommittee of the American Academy of Neurology, "Practice Parameters," 1016–1017.

[29] "Reliable criteria do not exist for making a diagnosis of PVS in infants under three months old, except in patients with anencephaly. Other diagnostic studies may support the diagnosis of PVS, but none adds to diagnostic specificity with certainty." Quality Standards Subcommittee of the American Academy of Neurology, "Practice Parameters," 1016.

[30] "Emerging Scientific Knowledge about Minimally Conscious States," 5.

[31] Ethics and Humanities Subcommittee of the American Academy of Neurology, "Certain Aspects of Care and Management of Profoundly and Irreversibly Paralyzed Patients with Retained Consciousness and Cognition."

[32] Multi-Society Task Force on PVS, "Medical Aspects of the Persistent Vegetative State—First of Two Parts."

[33] Ibid.; Jennett, *The Vegetative State: Medical Facts, Ethical and Legal Dilemmas.*

[34] Quality Standards Subcommittee of the American Academy of Neurology, "Practice Parameters."

[35] Ibid.

[36] Jennett, *The Vegetative State*, 60.

[37] Ibid., 61–62.

[38] For a more detailed analysis of data on recovery from a persistent vegetative state, see ibid., 57–72.

[39] Quality Standards Subcommittee of the American Academy of Neurology, "Practice Parameters."

[40] Multi-Society Task Force of the American Academy of Neurology, "Medical Aspects of the Persistent Vegetative State—Second of Two Parts."

[41] Ibid.

[42] Haig and Ruess, "Recovery from Vegetative State of Six Months' Duration Associated with Sinemet (levodopa/carbidopa)."

[43] Multi-Society Task Force of the American Academy of Neurology, "Medical Aspects of the Persistent Vegetative State—Second of Two Parts."

[44] Ibid.

[45] Doig and Burgess, 728. See also Younger et al., "'Brain Death' and Organ Retrieval: A Cross Sectional Survey and Concepts among Health Professionals."

[46] Rubenstein, Cohen, and Jackson, "The Definition of Death," 28.

TWO: ORDINARY VERSUS EXTRAORDINARY MEANS: THE ISSUE OF TUBE FEEDINGS

[1] John Paul II, "Care for Patients in a Persistent Vegetative State," 739.

[2] Ibid., 740.

[3] Sulmasy, "Are Feeding Tubes Morally Obligatory?" 2.

[4] Atkinson, "Theological History of Catholic Teaching on Prolonging Life."

[5] Aquinas, *Summa Theologica*.

[6] The *Relectio* was a lecture that De Vitoria, the preeminent theologian at the University of Salamanca, Spain, would give at the beginning of each school year. These lectures treated some difficult, contemporary dilemma. One can presume that the question of prolonging life must have been a disputed topic at the time.

[7] De Vitoria, "Relectio IX: de Temperentia."

[8] Ibid.; Sparks, *To Treat or Not to Treat*, 95.

[9] De Vitoria, "Relectio IX: de Temperentia"; Sparks, *To Treat or Not to Treat*, 94–95.

[10] Sparks, *To Treat or Not to Treat*, 96.

[11] Soto, *De Justitia et Jure*, Lib. 5, question 2, article 1; see also Sparks, *To Treat or Not to Treat*, 96.

[12] Wildes, "Ordinary and Extraordinary Means and the Quality of Life," 504.

[13]. Bañez, *Scholastica Commentaria in Partem Angelici Doctoris S. Thomae IV*, "Decisiones de Jure et Justitia," II, II ae, question 65, article 1. (Duaci: 1614–1615).

[14] Paris and McCormick, "The Catholic Tradition on the Use of Nutrition and Fluids," 358.

[15] De Lugo, "Disputationum de Justitia et Jure."

[16] Kelly, *Medico-Moral Problems*, 129.

[17] Kelly, "The Duty of Using Artificial Means of Preserving Life."

[18]. Cronin, *The Moral Law in Regard to Ordinary and Extraordinary Means of Conserving Life*; Paris and McCormick, "The Catholic Tradition on the Use of Nutrition and Fluids," 360.

[19] Pius XII, "Prolongation of Life."

[20] Wildes, "Ordinary and Extraordinary Means and the Quality of Life," 512.

[21] Pius XII, "Cancer: A Medical and Social Problem," *The Pope Speaks* 3 (1957): 48.

[22] Wildes, "Ordinary and Extraordinary Means and the Quality of Life," 512.

[23] Sacred Congregation for the Doctrine of the Faith, "Declaration on Euthanasia."

[24] Ibid.

²⁵ Ibid.

²⁶ Ibid.

²⁷ United States Catholic Conference of Bishops, *Ethical and Religious Directives for Catholic Health Care Services*, part 6.

²⁸ Ibid., #58.

²⁹ United States Catholic Conference of Bishops, *Ethical and Religious Directives for Catholic Health Care Services*, #58.

³⁰ John Paul II, "Care for Patients in a Persistent Vegetative State," 739.

³¹ Walter and Shannon, "Implications of the Papal Allocution on Tube Feeding," 19.

³² Hamel and Panicola, "Must We Preserve Life?" 9.

³³ Sheehan, "Feeding Tubes: Sorting Out the Issues," 23–24.

³⁴ Hamel and Panicola, "Must We Preserve Life?" 9.

³⁵ John Paul II, *Evangelium Vitae*, no. 65.

³⁶ Ibid.

³⁷ Shannon and Walter, "Artificial Nutrition, Hydration: Assessing Papal Statement," 2.

³⁸ Hamel and Panicola, "Must We Preserve Life?" 12.

³⁹ Shannon and Walter, "Artificial Nutrition, Hydration," 3.

⁴⁰ Hamel and Panicola, "Must We Preserve Life?" 9.

⁴¹ Lynn and Childress, "Must Patients Always Be Given Food and Water?"

⁴² Sacred Congregation for the Doctrine of the Faith, "Declaration on Euthanasia."

⁴³ Panicola, "Catholic Teaching on Prolonging Life: Setting the Record Straight," 17.

⁴⁴ Place, "Thoughts on the Papal Allocution."

⁴⁵ Ibid., 6.

⁴⁶ Walter and Shannon, "Implications of the Papal Allocution on Tube Feeding," 19; O'Rourke and Boyle, "Tissue Transplantation."

⁴⁷ John Paul II, *Evangelium Vitae,* no. 65.

⁴⁸ Gula, *Reason Informed by Faith*, 152–162.

⁴⁹ Hamel and Panicola, "Must We Preserve Life?" 12.

⁵⁰ Ibid.

⁵¹ Texas Catholic Bishops and the Texas Conference of Catholic Health Care Facilities, "On Withdrawing Artificial Nutrition and Hydration."

⁵² Dulles, "Authority and Conscience."

⁵³ Panicola, "Catholic Teaching on Prolonging Life: Setting the Record Straight," 15–16.

THREE: MEDICAL FUTILITY

¹ *Cruzan v. Director, Missouri Department of Health*; see also Jonsen, Veatch, and Walters, *Source Book in Bioethics: A Documentary History*, 229–237.

[2] Hippocrates, "On the Art," 193.

[3] In medical futility cases, the patient or surrogate wants to pursue the goal of preserving life even if there is little chance or no hope of future improvement, while the other party, the physician, sees dying as inevitable and wishes to pursue the goal of comfort care. For a more detailed analysis, see Council on Ethical and Judicial Affairs, American Medical Association, "Medical Futility in End-of-Life Care."

[4] The two prominent cases here would be the Helga Wanglie case and the Baby K case. For a more detailed analysis of both cases, see *In re Helen Wanglie*, Fourth Judicial District (District Court Probate Court Division) PX-91-238, Minnesota, Hennepin County; and *In re Baby K*, 16 F. 3d 590, petition for rehearing en banc denied, no. 93–1899 (L), CA-93-68-A, 28 March 1994. It should be noted that in the Wanglie case the court never addressed the question of whether physicians or the medical center could refuse to provide requested treatment, and thus, the conflict between nonmaleficence and beneficence and autonomy was not resolved. The court ruled that Mr. Wanglie should be appointed his wife's conservator on the grounds that he could best represent his wife's interests. In the Baby K case, physicians and ethics committees argued in Virginia that providing certain treatments such as mechanical ventilation to an anencephalic newborn was "futile" and "would serve no therapeutic or palliative purpose," and was "medically and ethically inappropriate." The courts ruled against them.

[5] Council on Ethical and Judicial Affairs, "Medical Futility in End-of-Life Care," 938.

[6] Brody and Halevy, "Is Futility a Futile Concept?" 124.

[7] Drane and Coulehan, "The Concept of Futility," 31. See also, Trau and McCartney, "In the Best Interest of the Patient."

[8] Schneiderman, Jecker, and Jonsen, "Medical Futility: Its Meaning and Ethical Implications."

[9] Fine and Mayo, "Resolution of Futility by Due Process: Early Experience with the Texas Advance Directive Act," 744; Texas Health and Safety Code 166.046 (a) (Vernon Supp 2002), accessed at www.capitol.state.tx.us/statutes/he/he00116600.html#he025.166.046 on February 5, 2007.

[10] "Baby at Center of Life-Support Battle Dies," *MSNBC*.

[11] The Health Care Quality Improvement Act requires professional liability insurers to report payments made on behalf of physicians to the National Practitioner Data Bank provided the payment is $10,000.00 or greater. See U.S.C.S., 11131–11137.

[12] *In re Wanglie*, No. PX-91-283 (Minn. Dist. Ct., Probate Ct. Div. July 1, 1991).

[13] *Gilgunn v. Massachusetts Hospital*, SUCV92-4820 (Massachusetts Superior Court, Suffolk County, April 21, 1995). See also Fine and Mayo, "Resolution of Futility by Due Process," 743.

[14] At the time, under Pennsylvania's Advance Directive for Health Care Act, a health care provider was required to comply with a patient's Advance Directive or transfer the patient to another provider. See 20 Pa. C.S.A. 5401-et seq.

[15] The Institutional Interdisciplinary Review Board (IIRB) is the Health Care System Board that will serve all four acute care facilities within the system in determining medical futility cases. The Board will consist of a physician, nurse, social worker, a representative of Mission Services, a pastoral care member, the bioethicist, and legal counsel. The Board will be appointed annually by the Senior Vice-President for Medical Affairs for the system. In addition, the Senior Vice-President for Medical Affairs will also appoint *ex officio* a physician from each specialty to serve as a consultant to the IIRB when appropriate.

[16] "Futility," in *The Oxford English Dictionary* Vol. IV (Oxford: Oxford University Press, 1989).

[17] Council on Ethical and Judicial Affairs, *Code of Medical Ethics*, #2.035 at p. 13.

[18] Council on Ethical and Judicial Affairs, "Medical Futility in End-of-Life Care," 938.

[19] Drane and Coulehan, "The Concept of Futility," 29.

[20] Cranford, "Medical Futility: Transforming a Clinical Concept into Legal and Social Policies," 897.

[21] Brody and Halevy, "Is Futility a Futile Concept?" 127–128.

[22] Griener, "The Physician's Authority to Withhold Futile Treatment," 209.

[23] Cranford, "Medical Futility: Transforming a Clinical Concept into Legal and Social Policies," 895.

[24] Schneiderman, Jecker, and Jonsen, "Medical Futility: Response to Critiques," 672. The authors go on to say, "In our experience, requests for futile treatment often represent not an appeal to respect the patient's wishes but rather a misguided effort to express caring for a patient by meeting a perceived duty to 'do everything' when other manifestations of devotion (such as comfort care) would be more appropriate." Ibid.

[25] Pellegrino, "Christ, Physician and Patient, the Model for Christian Healing," 75.

[26] Drane and Coulehan, "The Concept of Futility," 31.

[27] Grant, "Medical Futility: Legal and Ethical Aspects," 334.

[28] In recent years, a number of prognostic scoring systems have been developed to assist physicians in determining which patients are most likely to benefit from life-sustaining treatment. These systems, which include the Acute Physiology and Chronic Health Evaluation (APACHE) system, use databases to predict the hospital mortality of patients who receive critical care. Depending on the decision criteria used, the systems have positive predictive value of 80 percent, and a negative predictive value of 90 percent. These values correlate well with clinical judgment in most cases. Luce, "Physicians Do Not Have a Responsibility to Provide Futile or Unreasonable Care If a Patient or Family Insists," 761. See also, Schnei-

derman, Jecker, and Jonsen, "Medical Futility: Its Meaning and Ethical Implications."

[29] Pellegrino, "Christ, Physician and Patient, the Model for Christian Healing," 75.

[30] Drane and Coulehan, "The Concept of Futility," 29.

[31] Council on Ethical and Judicial Affairs, "Medical Futility in End-of-Life Care," 938.

[32] Jecker and Schneiderman, "Futility and Rationing," 195.

[33] Luce, "Physicians Do Not Have a Responsibility to Provide Futile or Unreasonable Care If a Patient or Family Insists," 764.

[34] Ibid.

[35] According to ethicist Gerald Kelly, S.J., and his classic interpretation of the ordinary–extraordinary means distinction in the Catholic tradition, "*ordinary* means of preserving life are all medicines, treatments, and operations, which offer a reasonable hope of benefit for the patient and which can be obtained and used without excessive expense, pain, or other inconvenience, *Extraordinary* means are all medicines, treatments, and operations, which cannot be obtained or used without excessive expense, pain, or other inconvenience, or which, if used, would not offer a reasonable hope of benefit." Kelly, *Medico-Moral Problems*, 129.

[36] Pius XII, "The Prolongation of Life," 395.

[37] Sacred Congregation for the Doctrine of the Faith, "Declaration on Euthanasia," 155.

[38] For a more detailed analysis of the Houston Policy, see Halevy and Brody, "The Houston Process-Based Approach to Medical Futility."

[39] Drane and Coulehan, "The Concept of Futility," 32.

FOUR: "DO NOT RESUSCITATE" ORDERS, LIVING WILLS/ADVANCE DIRECTIVES, AND DURABLE POWERS OF ATTORNEY FOR HEALTH CARE

[1] President's Council on Bioethics. *Taking Care: Ethical Caregiving in Our Aging Society*, chapter 1; *Older Americans 2004: Key Indicators of Well-Being*.

[2] Lynn, *Sick to Death and Not Going to Take It Anymore!*, 21.

[3] Miller, "Making Decisions about Advance Health Care Directives," 91.

[4] Task Force for Quality at the End of Life, "Improving End-of-Life Experiences for Pennsylvanians."

[5] Vitz, "Let Us Not Forsake the Dying, Says Pa. Report," 1.

[6] "MCW Researchers Identify Steps to Improve CPR Survival," 1.

[7] "Do Not Resuscitate Orders."

[8] Ringold and Glass, "Cardiopulmonary Resuscitation (CPR)."

[9] Wik et al., "Quality of Cardiopulmonary Resuscitation During Out-of-Hospital Cardiac Arrest"; Abella et al., "Quality of Cardiopulmonary Resuscitation During In-Hospital Cardiac Arrest."

[10] Hazinski et al., "Major Changes in 2005 AHA Guidelines for CPR and ECC."

[11] Christopoulos, "Doctors Hope to Push CPR to New Level," 1.

[12] Brindley et al., "Predictors of Survival Following In-Hospital Adult Cardiopulmonary Resuscitation," 2.

[13] Ibid., 2–3.

[14] The drugs used in cardiac arrest depend on what rhythm the patient is in at that moment. If in asystole, the drug of choice is epinephrine; for bradycardia, it is atropine; for ventricular tachycardia, lidocaine. Among other approved medications are procainamide and amiodarone.

[15] "The Slow Code—Should Anyone Rush to Its Defense?" 467.

[16] Cohen, "A Tale of Two Conversations."

[17] Ibid, 49.

[18] Pennsylvania Department of Health. "Out-of-Hospital Do-Not-Resuscitate (DNR) Orders: A Guide for Patients and Families," 1.

[19] Miller, "Making Decisions about Advance Health Care Directives," 92.

[20] United States Congress, "Federal Patient Self-Determination Act of 1990."

[21] Shaw, "POLST: Honoring Wishes at the End of Life," 8. See also SUPPORT Principle Investigators, "A Controlled Trial to Improve Care for Seriously Ill Hospitalized Patients: A Study to Understand Prognoses and Preferences for Outcomes and Risks of Treatments (SUPPORT)."

[22] "Do Not Resuscitate Orders," 3.

[23] Miller, "Making Decisions about Advance Health Care Directives," 97–98.

[24] Pennsylvania Legislature, "Act 169 of 2006—Pennsylvania Health Care Decision Making."

[25] Ibid., section 5442.

[26] Miller, "Making Decisions about Advance Health Care Directives," 100.

[27] Ibid., 101–106.

[28] Pennsylvania Legislature, "Act 169 of 2006—Pennsylvania Health Care Decision Making," sections 5443–5446. See also Pennsylvania Medical Society. "Advance Health Care Directives and Health Care Decision-Making for Incompetent Patients: A Guide to Act 169 of 2006 for Physicians and Other Health Care Providers," 11.

[29] Pennsylvania Legislature, "Act 169 of 2006," section 5444; Pennsylvania Medical Society, "A Guide to Act 169 of 2006," 2–3.

[30] Pennsylvania Medical Society, "A Guide to Act 169 of 2006," 1.

[31] Shaw, "POLST: Honoring Wishes at the End of Life," 8.

[32] Ibid. See also Tolle et al., "A Prospective Study of the Efficacy of the Physician Order Form for Life-Sustaining Treatment."

[33] Pennsylvania Legislature, "Act 169 of 2006," sections 5452–5455; Pennsylvania Medical Society, "A Guide to Act 169 of 2006," 1.

[34] "Five Wishes," *Aging With Dignity*.

[35] Pennsylvania Medical Society, "A Guide to Act 169 of 2006," 3–5.

[36] Miller, "Making Decisions about Advance Health Care Directives," 98.

[37] Pennsylvania Medical Society, "A Guide to Act 169 of 2006," 3; Pennsylvania Legislature, "Act 169 of 2006," section 5456.

[38] Pennsylvania Medical Society, "A Guide to Act 169 of 2006," 3–6; Pennsylvania Legislature, "Act 169 of 2006," section 5459.

[39] Pennsylvania Medical Society, "A Guide to Act 169 of 2006," 6–8.

[40] Ibid., 8–10.

[41] Pennsylvania Legislature, "Act 169 of 2006," subchapter C, sections 5451–5465.

[42] Lynn and Adamson, "Living Well at the End of Life: Adapting Health Care to Serious Chronic Illness in Old Age," 18.

FIVE: PAIN MANAGEMENT

[1] Meldrum, "A Capsule History of Pain Management," 2470.

[2] Ibid.

[3] Ibid., 2471; see also Ballantyne and Mao, "Opioid Therapy for Chronic Pain."

[4] Meldrum, "A Capsule History of Pain Management," 2470–2471.

[5] Ibid., 2474.

[6] Ibid.

[7] Hippocrates, "The Art."

[8] Council on Ethical and Judicial Affairs, *Code of Medical Ethics*, 2:20.

[9] SUPPORT Principal Investigators, "A Controlled Trial."

[10] Lynn et al., "Perceptions by Family Members of the Dying Experience of Older and Seriously Ill Patients."

[11] Institute of Medicine, *Approaching Death: Improving Care at the End of Life.*

[12] Schnitzer, "Non-NSAID Pharmacologic Treatment Options for the Management of Chronic Pain."

[13] Satel, "Doctors Behind Bars: Treating Pain Is Now Risky Business," 1.

[14] Teno, et al., "Research Letter: Persistent Pain in Nursing Home Residents."

[15] Bernabei et al., "Management of Pain in Elderly Patients with Cancer."

[16] Ferrell, Ferrell, and Rivera, "Pain in Cognitively Impaired Nursing Home Patients"; and Sengstaken and King, "The Problems of Pain and Its Detection among Geriatric Nursing Home Residents."

17 Rich "An Ethical Analysis of the Barriers to Effective Pain Management." See also Marks and Sachar, "Undertreatment of Medical Inpatients with Narcotic Analgesics."

[18] Joint Commission on Accreditation of Healthcare Organizations, *Comprehensive Accreditation Manual for Hospitals: The Official Handbook.*

[19] Foley, "Controlling Cancer Pain."

[20] Jenkins et al., "Opioid Prescribing: An Assessment Using Quality Statements."

[21]. *Washington v. Glucksberg*, 65 *U.S. Law Wk.* 4669, 117 S. Ct. 2258 (1997); *Vacco v. Quill*, 65 *U.S. Law Wk.* 4695, 117 S. Ct. 2293 (1997).

[22] Justice Sandra Day O'Connor opined that those individuals suffering from a terminal illness accompanied with great pain may currently obtain whatever level of medication determined professionally by a physician will "alleviate that suffering, even to the point of causing unconsciousness and hastening death." See note 21, *Washington v. Glucksberg*, at 4679; *Vacco v. Quill*, at 4700. Justice John Paul Stevens concluded that since palliative care cannot alleviate every degree of pain and suffering for all patients, there may be situations in which a competent person could make an informed judgment or "a rational choice for assisted suicide." See note 21, *Washington v. Glucksberg*, at 4682; *Vacco v. Quill*, at 4703. Also see Angell, "The Supreme Court and Physician-Assisted Suicide—The Ultimate Right."

[23] The most recent case was that of *Tomlinson v. Bayberry Care Center* in 2003. Charges of inadequate pain management were brought successfully against both the treating physician and the patient's nursing home. Quill and Meier, "The Big Chill: Inserting the DEA into End-of-Life Care." In another case, *Bergman v. Chin*, the family of William Bergman sued his physician Dr. Wing Chin for undertreating Mr. Bergman's pain. The family argued that their father was denied proper pain medication during a five-day stay at Eden Medical Center in Castro Valley, California, where he was admitted in February 1998, complaining of intolerable back pain. During the course of his hospital stay, nurses charted Mr. Bergman's pain levels ranging from 7 to 10 on a scale that awards a 10 to the worst pain imaginable. Mr. Bergman was discharged and died of lung cancer at home three days later under the care of a hospice program. On June 13, 2001, an Alameda County jury awarded $1.5 million to the family of William Bergman. The jury found Dr. Wing Chin guilty of elder abuse and recklessness for failure to give a dying man sufficient medication to relieve his suffering. The jury deadlocked on whether Dr. Chin was guilty of malice, oppression, or intentional emotional distress. The family settled its suit against the Eden Medical Center in Castro Valley, California on May 7, 2001 before the trial began. As part of the settlement, the hospital has agreed to provide pain management classes to its staff and to physicians who admit patients to the hospital. See LaGanga and Monmaney, "Doctor Found Liable in Suit over Pain"; Okie, "Doctor's Duty to Ease Pain at Issue in California Lawsuit." There had been two previous lawsuits for the undertreatment of pain that resulted in large damage awards. A North Carolina jury awarded $15 million in damages in a 1990 lawsuit against a nursing home where a nurse failed to administer prescribed pain medicine to a terminally ill patient. See, *Estate of Henry James v. Hillhaven Corp.*, 89 CVS 64 (S.C. Hertford County, North Carolina, 1991). A judge in a 1997 case in South Carolina awarded $200,000 in damages for pain and suffering caused by inadequate treatment of a cancer patient's pain.

[24] Rich, "An Ethical Analysis of the Barriers to Effective Pain Management," 55.

[25] Merskey and Bogduk, eds., *Classification of Chronic Pain*, xi.

[26] Sternbach, "Clinical Aspects of Pain."

[27] Recent research suggests that infants may be more vulnerable to the negative effects of pain, which may later affect their neurological development, including the reaction to pain. See, Larsson, "Pain Management in Neonates."

[28] Cutson, "Management of Cancer Pain."

[29] Berkow and Beers, eds., *The Merck Manual of Diagnosis and Therapy*, 1363.

[30] Quill and Meier, "The Big Chill," 1.

[31] Effective pain management has been shown to shorten hospital stays and reduce costs. For a more detailed analysis, see Slack and Faut-Callahan, "Pain Management."

[32] Stewart et al., "Lost Productive Time and Cost Due to Common Pain Conditions in the US Workforce."

[33] Rich, "An Ethical Analysis of the Barriers to Effective Pain Management," 54.

[34] Task Force on Pain Management, Catholic Health Association, "Pain Management: Theological and Ethical Principles Governing the Use of Pain Relief for Dying Patients," *Health Progress* (January–February 1993): 30–39, 65.

[35] Rich, "An Ethical Analysis of the Barriers to Effective Pain Management," 56.

[36] DeAngelis, "Pain Management," 2480.

[37] Donovan and Miaskowski, "Striving for a Standard of Pain Relief."

[38] Rich, "An Ethical Analysis of the Barriers to Effective Pain Management," 56.

[39] Rich, "Pain Management: Legal Risks and Ethical Responsibilities."

[40] For a more detailed analysis of this topic, see Weiner, "An Interview with John J. Bonica, M.D."

[41] Hill, "When Will Adequate Pain Treatment Be the Norm?'

[42] Rich, "An Ethical Analysis of the Barriers to Effective Pain Management," 9.

[43] Ibid., 54.

[44] Ibid., 60. The one state medical board that did discipline a physician for not adequately managing a patient's pain was Oregon. See, "*Foubister v. Oregon*: Doctor Cited for Negligence for Undertreating Pain."

[45] Quill and Meier, "The Big Chill," 2–3.

[46] "Top Court OKs Assisted-Suicide Law."

[47] Rich, "An Ethical Analysis of the Barriers to Effective Pain Management," 60.

[48] Satel, "Doctors Behind Bars," 2.

[49] Rich, "An Ethical Analysis of the Barriers to Effective Pain Management," 63.

[50] Ibid., 54.

[51] Porter and Jick, "Addiction Rare in Patients Treated with Narcotics."

[52] Rich, "An Ethical Analysis of the Barriers to Effective Pain Management," 64.

[53] Satel, "Doctors Behind Bars," 2.

[54] "New Medication for Cancer Breakthrough Pain," 1.

[55] Ibid.

[56] Ibid.

[57] Rich, "An Ethical Analysis of the Barriers to Effective Pain Management," 65. See also Agency of Health Care Policy and Research, *Management of Cancer Pain*, 61–65.

[58] National Commission for the Protection of Human Subjects of Biomedical and Behavioral Research, *The Belmont Report: Ethical Principles and Guidelines for the Protection of Human Subjects of Research*, B-1.

[59] Pellegrino and Thomasma, *A Philosophical Basis of Medical Practice*, 213.

[60] Rich, "An Ethical Analysis of the Barriers to Effective Pain Management," 62.

[61] Ferrell, "Cost Issues Surrounding the Treatment of Cancer Related Pain."

[62] Illinois Bishops, "Facing the End of Life."

[63] National Conference of Catholic Bishops, *Ethical and Religious Directives for Catholic Health Care Services*, # 61, at p. 28, 5th Edition.

[64] Ibid.

[65] For a more detailed analysis, see Kelly, *Medico-Moral Problems*, 12–16.

[66] Berkow, ed., *The Merck Manual of Diagnosis and Therapy*, 16th ed., 1409–1410.

[67] Ibid., 1410.

[68] Mangan, "An Historical Analysis of the Principle of Double Effect," 41.

[69] For further analysis on the historical development of the principle of double effect, see Kaczor, "Double-Effect Reasoning from Jean Pierre Gury to Peter Knauer"; Cavanaugh, "Aquinas' Account of Double Effect"; Keenan, "The Function of the Principle of Double Effect"; and Boyle, "Double Effect and a Certain Kind of Embryotomy."

[70] Kelly, *Medico-Moral Problems*, 13–14.

[71] For a more detailed description of the proportionalist's argument, see Keenan, "The Function of the Principle of Double Effect," 301–302; Knauer, "*La détermination du bien et du mal moral par le principe de double effet*"; Katchadourian, "Is the Principle of Double Effect Morally Acceptable?"; Cornerotte, "*Loi morale, valeurs humaines et situations de conflit*"; Hoose, *Proportionalism: The American Debate and Its European Roots*; Schüller, "The Double Effect in Catholic Thought: A Reevaluation"; and McCormick, *Notes on Moral Theology: 1965 through 1980*, 751–756.

[72] Walter, "Proportionate Reason and Its Three Levels of Inquiry: Structuring the Ongoing Debate," 32.

[73] McCormick's criteria for proportionate reason first appeared in McCormick, *Ambiguity in Moral Choice*. He later reworked the criteria in response to criticism. His revised criteria can be found in McCormick and Ramsey, eds., *Doing Evil to Achieve Good*.

[74] Grady, "Medical and Ethical Questions Raised on Deaths of Critically Ill Patients."

[75] Jansen and Sulmasy, "Sedation, Alimentation, Hydration, and Equivocation: Careful Conversation about Care at the End of Life," 845; see also Barilan, "Terminal Sedation, Terminal Elation, and Medical Parsimony."

[76] Jansen and Sulamsy, "Sedation, Alimentation, Hydration, and Equivocation," 845.

[77] Ibid., 847.

[78] Trafford, "No Pain Relief for Some: Study Points Out Inequality in Care."

[79] A simple 0–10 numeric scale that rates pain from "none" to "worst imaginable" and pain relief from "none" to "total" can be used with most patients over seven years of age. Patients should be shown the scale and should be asked about pain intensity on admission, after each painful procedure, and at least once per shift. With children under seven years of age (and with the cognitively impaired) the same type scale can be used but with faces.

[80] Quill and Meier, "The Big Chill," 2.

[81] Satel, "Doctors Behind Bars," 3.

[82] Hampton, "Researchers Probe Pathways of Pain," 2391.

[83] Vastag, "Scientists Find Connections in the Brain between Physical and Emotional Pain," 2389.

[84] Hampton, "Researchers Probe Pathways of Pain," 2392.

[85] DeAngelis, "Pain Management," 2481.

SIX: PALLIATIVE CARE AND HOSPICE

[1] Cousins, *Anatomy of an Illness as Perceived by the Patient: Reflections on Healing and Regeneration*, 133.

[2] Morrison and Meier, "Palliative Care," 2582.

[3] "Hospice Facts and Statistics," 1–11. http://www.nahc.org/Consumer/hpc-stats.html.

[4] Morrison and Meier, "Palliative Care," 2583.

[5] World Health Organization, "Definition of Palliative Care."

[6] "What is Hospice?" 1.

[7] Taylor, "Hospice: Caring When There Is No Cure."

[8] Mayo Clinic Staff, "Hospice Care: An Option for People with Terminal Illness," 1. http//www.mayoclinic.com/health/hospice-care/HQ00860.

[9] Meldrum, "A Capsule History of Pain Management," 2473–2474.

[10] "Hospice Facts and Statistics," 1.

[11] Ibid., 2.

[12] Center to Advance Palliative Care, "A Guide to Building a Hospital-Based Palliative Care Program."

[13] "NHPCO's Facts and Figures—2005 Findings," 1.

[14] Morrison and Meier, "Palliative Care," 2586.

[15] Ackerman, "Goldilocks and Mrs. Ilych: A Critical Look at the 'Philosophy of Hospice,'" 314; and Manard and Perrone, *Hospice Care: An Introduction and Review of Evidence*, 4.

[16] National Hospice and Palliative Care Organization, *Hospice Care: A Physician's Guide*, 9.

[17] Ibid., 10–11.

[18] Ibid., 11.

[19] National Hospice and Palliative Care Organization (NPHCO), "Facts and Figures—2005 Findings" (November 2006): 1–3.

[20] Banerjee, "A Place to Turn When a Newborn Is Fated to Die."

[21] "Hospice, Palliative and End of Life Statistics," 1; and Abelson "A Chance to Pick Hospice, and Still Hope to Live," 1.

[22] In 1932 the United States Public Health Service initiated a study on African American men with syphilis in Macon County, Alabama, to determine the natural course of untreated, latent syphilis in black males. The study comprised 399 syphilitic men as well as 201 uninfected men who served as the control group. These subjects were recruited from churches and clinics throughout Macon County and were led to believe they would receive free meals, "special free treatment" for what was called "bad blood," and burial insurance. In reality, they were enrolled in this study without informed consent. These men were deceived in that the infected were never told they had syphilis, which was known to cause mental illness and death. In fact, the infected were never treated for the disease. To determine the natural course of syphilis, the researchers withheld the standard treatment of mercury and arsenic compounds from the subjects. In 1947, when penicillin was determined to be an effective treatment for syphilis, this too was withheld. The treatment these men actively received came in the form of placebos. The Tuskegee Syphilis Study was a covert medical research study. It was widely known in medical circles due to published articles in major medical journals. As late as 1969, a committee at the federally operated CDC examined the study and agreed to allow it to continue. Not until 1972, when the first accounts of this study appeared in the press, did the Department of Health, Education and Welfare (HEW) terminate the experiment. At that time, seventy-four of the test subjects were still alive; at least twenty-eight, but perhaps more than one hundred, had died directly from advanced syphilitic lesions. For a more detailed analysis, see Allen "Racism and Research: The Case of the Tuskegee Syphilis Study"; and Ad Hoc Advisory Panel, Department of Health, Education and Welfare, "Final Report of the Tuskegee Syphilis Study." Caplan, "When Evil Intrudes"; Harold, "Outside the Community"; King,

"The Dangers of Difference"; Jones, "The Tuskegee Legacy: AIDS and the Black Community"; and Jones, *Bad Blood: The Tuskegee Syphilis Experiment—A Tragedy of Race and Medicine.*

[23] Waldman, "A Last Compassion Resisted."

[24] "NHPCO's Facts and Figures," 3.

[25] "Hospice Facts and Statistics," 2–3.

[26] Ibid., 4.

[27] Ibid., 3.

[28] Ibid., 7. See also, Kidder, "The Effects of Hospice Coverage on Medicare Expenditures."

[29] Abelson, "A Chance to Pick Hospice, and Still Hope to Live."

[30] "Hospice Fact Sheet," 2–3.

[31] Mayo Clinic Staff, "Hospice Care," 3.

[32] Ackerman, "Goldilocks and Mrs. Ilych," 315–321

[33] Ibid., 315–321.

[34] Mulvihill, "Giving Patients a 'Good Death.'"

[35] Morrison and Meier, "Palliative Care," 2586. See also Christakis and Iwashyna, "The Health Impact of Health Care on Families: A Matched Cohort Study of Hospice Use by Decedents and Mortality Outcomes in Surviving, Widowed Spouses"; and Teno et al., "Family Perspectives on End-of-Life Care at the Last Place of Care."

[36] "Hospice Facts and Statistics," 11.

Seven: Spirituality and End-of-Life Care

[1] McCormick, "To Save or Let Die: The Dilemma of Modern Medicine," 345.

[2] Lo et al., "Discussing Religious and Spiritual Issues at the End of Life," 749.

[3] Sulmasy, *The Healer's Calling: A Spirituality for Physicians and Other Health Care Professionals*, 10.

[4] Gula, "Spirituality and Ethics in Healthcare," 17.

[5] Sulmasy, *The Healer's Calling*, 13.

[6] Ibid., 12.

[7] Ibid., 13.

[8] Ibid.

[9] Olive, "Religion and Spirituality: Important Variables Frequently Ignored in Clinical Research."

[10] Modjarrad, "Medicine and Spirituality."

[11] O'Hara, "Is There a Role for Prayer and Spirituality in Health Care?" 33. See also Eliade, *The Sacred and the Profane*; Marrone, "Dying, Mourning and Spirituality: A Psychological Perspective."

[12] O'Hara, "Is There a Role for Prayer and Spirituality in Health Care?" 35–36. See also Galton, "Statistical Inquiries into the Efficacy of Prayer."

[13] O'Hara, "Is There a Role for Prayer and Spirituality in Health Care?" 36. See also Gartner, Larson, and Allen, "Religious Commitment and Mental Health: A Review of the Empirical Literature."

[14] O'Hara, "Is There a Role for Prayer and Spirituality in Health Care?" 38–39. See also Byrd, "Positive Therapeutic Effects of Intercessory Prayer in a Coronary Care Unit Population."

[15] Wirth and Mitchell, "Complementary Healing Therapy for Patients with Type-1 Diabetes Milletus."

[16] Carey, "Can Prayer Heal? Critics Say Studies Go Past Science's Reach."

[17] Benson et al., "Study of the Therapeutic Effects of Intercessory Prayer in Cardiac Bypass Patients: A Multicenter Randomized Trial of Uncertainty and Certainty of Receiving Intercessory Prayer."

[18] Ibid., 934.

[19] Carey "Long-Awaited Medical Study Questions the Power of Prayer," 2.

[20] Ibid., 1.

[21] O'Hara, "Is There a Role for Prayer and Spirituality in Health Care?" 42.

[22] McCaffrey et al., "Prayer for Health Concerns," 861.

[23] Ellis and Campbell, "Patients' Views about Discussing Spiritual Issues with Primary Care Physicians," 1163.

[24] O'Hara, "Is There a Role for Prayer and Spirituality in Health Care?" 42–43.

[25] Ibid., 34. See also Poloma and Pendleton, "The Effects of Prayer and Prayer Experiences on Measures of General Well-Being."

[26] Sulmasy, *The Healer's Calling*, 15.

[27] Ellis and Campbell, "Patients' Views," 1161.

[28] Ibid., 1162–1163.

[29] Curlin et al., "Physicians' Observations and Interpretations of the Influence of Religion and Spirituality on Health," 649.

[30] Lo et al., "Discussing Religious and Spiritual Issues at the End of Life," 749. See also, Sloan, Bagiella, and Powell, "Religion, Spirituality, and Medicine," and Cohen, Wheeler, and Scott, "Walking a Fine Line: Physician Inquiries Into Patient's Religious and Spiritual Beliefs."

[31] Lo et al., "Discussing Religious and Spiritual Issues at the End of Life," 749.

[32] Ibid., 750.

[33] Ibid., 751.

[34] Ibid., 753.

[35] Ibid., 749.

[36] Daly, "Religion and the Attending Physician's Point-of-View," *Southern Medical Journal* 98, 8 (August 2005): 759.

[37] McCormick, *Corrective Vision: Explorations in Moral Theology*, 145.

[38] McCormick, *Health and Medicine in the Catholic Tradition*, 116–117.

[39] Christiansen, "The Elderly and Their Families: The Problems of Dependence," 102.

[40] Ibid., 104.

[41] Ibid., 102.

[42] Kelleher, "Ritual."

[43] Joint Commission of Catholic Bishops' Conferences, "Order for the Blessing of Adults," 165.

[44] Clark, "The Transition between Ending Medical Treatment and Beginning Palliative Care: The Need for a Ritual Response," 350–353.

[45] Kuczewski, "Talking about Spirituality in the Clinical Setting: Can Being Professional Require Being Personal?" 18.

[46] McCaffrey et al., "Prayer for Health Concerns," 861.

EIGHT: CONCLUSION

[1] Landau and Gustafson, "Death Is Not the Enemy."

[2] Bernardin, A Sign of Hope, 5.

[3] Steinhauser et al., "In Search of a Good Death: Observations of Patients, Families, and Providers," 830.

[4] Sulmasy, The Healer's Calling, 103.

[5] Kalina, "Hope for the Journey: Meaningful Support for the Terminally Ill," 91.

[6] Emanuel et al., "Understanding Economic and Other Burdens of Terminal Illness: The Experience of Patients and Their Caregivers," 451.

[7] Council on Ethical and Juridical Affairs, Code of Medical Ethics, 279.

[8] Arnold and Egan, "Breaking the 'Bad' News to Patients and Families: Preparing to Have the Conversation about End-of-Life and Hospice Care," 307.

[9] Landau and Gustafson, "Death Is Not the Enemy," 2458.

BIBLIOGRAPHY

Abella, B., et al. "Quality of Cardiopulmonary Resuscitation during In-Hospital Cardiac Arrest." *Journal of the American Medical Association* 293 (January 19, 2005): 305–310.

Abelson, R. "A Chance to Pick Hospice, and Still Hope to Live." *New York Times* (February 10, 2007): 1–5. http://www.nytimes.com/2007/02/10/business/10hospice.html.

Ackerman, F. "Goldilocks and Mrs. Ilych: A Critical Look at the 'Philosophy of Hospice,'" *Cambridge Quarterly of Health Care Ethics* 6 (1997): 314–324.

Ad Hoc Advisory Panel, Department of Health, Education and Welfare. "Final Report of the Tuskegee Syphilis Study." Washington, DC: Government Printing Office, 1973.

Ad Hoc Committee of the Harvard Medical School to Examine the Definition of Brain Death. "A Definition of Irreversible Coma." *Journal of the American Medical Association* 205 (1968): 337–340.

Agency of Health Care Policy and Research, *Management of Cancer Pain*. Washington, DC: Agency of Health Care Policy and Research, 1994.

Allen, B. "Racism and Research: The Case of the Tuskegee Syphilis Study." *Hastings Center Report* 8 (December 1978): 21.

Angell, M. "The Supreme Court and Physician-Assisted Suicide—The Ultimate Right." *New England Journal of Medicine* 336 (1997): 50–53.

Aquinas, T. *Summa Theologica*. A. Ross and P. G. Walsh, eds. Blackfriars edition. New York: McGraw Hill, 1966.

Arnold, R., and K. Egan. "Breaking the 'Bad' News to Patients and Families: Preparing to Have the Conversation about End-of-Life and Hospice Care." *American Journal of Geriatric Cardiology* 13, no. 6 (2004): 307–312.

Atkinson, G. "Theological History of Catholic Teaching on Prolonging Life." In McCarthy, D., and A. Moraczewski eds., *Moral Responsibility in Prolonging Life Decisions*. St. Louis, MO: Pope John Center, 1981.

"Baby at Center of Life-Support Battle Dies." *MSNBC* (March 15, 2005): 1–3. http://www.msnbc.msn.com/id/7190468/.

Baile, W. F., et al. "SPIKES—A Six-Step Protocol for Delivering Bad News: Application to the Patient with Cancer." *The Oncologist* 5, no. 4 (August 2000): 1–15. http://theoncologist.alphamedpress.org/cgi/content/full/5/4/302.

Ballantyne, J., and J. Mao. "Opioid Therapy for Chronic Pain." *New England Journal of Medicine* 349 (2003): 1943–1953.

Banerjee, N. "A Place to Turn When a Newborn Is Fated to Die." *New York Times* (March 13, 2007): 1–6. http://www.nytimes.com/2007/03/13/health/13hospice.html?_r=1&th=&oref=slogin&emc.

Bañez, D. *Scholastica Commentaria in Partem Angelici Doctoris S. Thomae*. Duaci: 1614–1615.

Barilan, Y. M. "Terminal Sedation, Terminal Elation, and Medical Parsimony." *Ethics in Medicine* 20, no. 3 (2004): 151–165.

Benson, H., et al. "Study of the Therapeutic Effects of Intercessory Prayer in Cardiac Bypass Patients: A Multicenter Randomized Trial of Uncertainty and Certainty of Receiving Intercessory Prayer." *American Heart Journal* 151, no. 4 (April 2006): 934–942.

Berkow, R., ed. *The Merck Manual of Diagnosis and Therapy,* 16th ed. Rahway, NJ: Merck Research Laboratories, 1992.

———, and M. Beers, eds. *The Merck Manual of Diagnosis and Therapy*, 17th ed. Whitehouse Station, NJ: Merck Research Laboratories, 1999.

Bernabei, R., et al. (SAGE Study Group: Systematic Assessment of Geriatric Drug Use via Epidemiology). "Management of Pain in Elderly Patients with Cancer." *Journal of the American Medical Association* 279 (1998): 1877–1882.

Bernardin, B. *A Sign of Hope.* St. Louis, MO: Catholic Health Association, 1996.

Boyle, J. "Double Effect and a Certain Kind of Embryotomy." *Irish Theological Quarterly* 44 (1977): 303–318.

"Brain Death—Well Settled Yet Still Unresolved." *New England Journal of Medicine* 344, no. 16 (April 19, 2001): 1244–1246.

Brindley, P., et al. "Predictors of Survival Following In-Hospital Adult Cardiopulmonary Resuscitation." *Canadian Medical Association Journal* 167, no. 4 (2002): 1–9. http://www.cmaj.ca/cgi/content/full/167/4/343.

Brody, B., and A. Halevy. "Is Futility a Futile Concept?" *Journal of Medicine and Philosophy* 20 (April 1995): 123–144.

Byrd, R. C. "Positive Therapeutic Effects of Intercessory Prayer in a Coronary Care Unit Population." *Southern Medical Journal* 81 (1988): 826–829.

Caplan, A. "When Evil Intrudes." *Hastings Center Report* 22 (November–December 1992): 29–32.

Carey, B. "Can Prayer Heal? Critics Say Studies Go Past Science's Reach." *New York Times* (October 10, 2004): 1–4. http://www.nytimes.com /2004/10/10/health/10prayer.html.

———. "Long-Awaited Medical Study Questions the Power of Prayer." *New York Times* (March 31, 2006): 1–2.

Cavanaugh, T. "Aquinas' Account of Double Effect." *Thomist* 61 (1997): 107–121.

Center to Advance Palliative Care. "A Guide to Building a Hospital-Based Palliative Care Program" (2006). http://www.capc.org.

Christakis, N. A., and T. J. Iwashyna. "The Health Impact of Health Care on Families: A Matched Cohort Study of Hospice Use by Decedents and Mortality Outcomes in Surviving, Widowed Spouses." *Social Science Medicine* 57 (2003): 465–475.

Christiansen, D. "The Elderly and Their Families: The Problems of Dependence." *New Catholic World* 223 (1980): 102.

Christopoulos, K. "Doctors Hope to Push CPR to New Level." *New York Times* (March 15, 2005): 1–3. http://www.nytimes.com/2005/03/15/health/policy/15cpr.html?_r=1.

Clark, P. A. "Medical Futility in Pediatrics: Is It Time for a Public Policy?" *Journal of Public Health Policy* 23 (2002): 66–89.

———. "The Transition between Ending Medical Treatment and Beginning Palliative Care: The Need for a Ritual Response." *Worship* 72 (July 1998): 345–354.

———, and C. M. Mikus. "Medical Futility: Is It Time to Establish a Formalized Policy?" *Health Progress* 81 (July–August 2000): 24–32.

Cohen, C. B., S. E. Wheeler, and D. A. Scott. "Walking a Fine Line: Physician Inquiries into Patients' Religious and Spiritual Beliefs." *Hastings Center Report* 31 (2001): 29–39.

Cohen, R. "A Tale of Two Conversations." *Hastings Center Report* 34 (May–June 2004): 49.

Congregation for the Doctrine of the Faith. "Declaration on Euthanasia" Part IV, *Origins* 10 (1980): 154–157.

Cornerotte, L. "*Loi morale, valeurs humaines et situations de conflit.*" *Nouvelle revue Théologique* 100 (1978): 502–532.

Council on Ethical and Judicial Affairs. *Code of Medical Ethics: Current Opinions with Annotations*, 2004–2005 edition. Chicago, IL: American Medical Association, 1998–1999.

———. "Medical Futility in End-of-Life Care." *Journal of the American Medical Association* 281 (March 10, 1999): 937–941.

Cousins, N. *Anatomy of an Illness as Perceived by the Patient: Reflections on Healing and Regeneration.* New York: Norton, 1979.

Cranford, R. E. "Medical Futility: Transforming a Clinical Concept into Legal and Social Policies." *Journal of the American Geriatrics Society* 42 (1994): 894–898.

Crippen, D. "Brain Failure and Brain Death: Introduction." *ACS Surgery Online, Critical Care* (April 2005). http://www.acssurgery.com/abstracts/acs/acs0812.htm. Retrieved on January 9, 2007.

Cronin, D. *The Moral Law in Regard to Ordinary and Extraordinary Means of Conserving Life.* Rome: Gregorian, 1958.

Cruzan v. Director, Missouri Department of Health, 110 S. Ct. 2841 (1990).

Curlin, F., et al. "Physicians' Observations and Interpretations of the Influence of Religion and Spirituality on Health," *Archives of Internal Medicine* 167 (2007): 649–654.

Cutson, T. M. "Management of Cancer Pain." *Primary Care* 25 (1998): 407–421.

Daly, C. "Religion and the Attending Physician's Point-of-View." *Southern Medical Journal* 98, no. 8 (August 2005): 759.

DeAngelis, C. "Pain Management." *Journal of the American Medical Association* 290, no. 18 (November 12, 2003): 2480–2481

De Lugo, J. *"Disputationum de Justitia et Jure."* In *De Justitia et Jure* 10, sec. 1, n. 9 (Lyons: Gousset, 1642).

De Vitoria, F. "Relectio IX: de Temperentia." In *Relectiones Theologicae.* Lugdini: 1587. Cf. *Relecciones Theologicas*, edition critica. Madrid: Imprenta La Rafa, volume III, 1933–1935.

Doig, C., and E. Burgess. "Brain Death: Resolving Inconsistencies in the Ethical Declaration of Death." *Canadian Journal of Anesthesia* 50 (2003): 725–731. http://www.cja-jca.org/cgi/content/full/50/7/725.

"Do Not Resuscitate Orders." *Ethics in Medicine* (University of Washington School of Medicine, 1999): 1–4. http://eduserv.hscer.washington.edu/bioethics/topics/dnr.html.

Donovan, M. I., and C. Miaskowski. "Striving for a Standard of Pain Relief." *American Journal of Nursing* 92 (1992): 106–107.

Drane, J., and J. Coulehan. "The Concept of Futility." *Health Progress* 74 (December 1993): 28–32.

Dulles, A. "Authority and Conscience." In *Moral Theology No. 6: Dissent in the Church*. Mahwah, NJ: Paulist Press, 1988 (97–111).

Eliade, M. *The Sacred and the Profane*. New York: Harper & Brothers, 1957.

Ellis, M. R., and J. D. Campbell. "Patients' Views about Discussing Spiritual Issues with Primary Care Physicians." *Southern Medical Journal* 97, no. 12 (December 2004): 1158–1164.

Emanuel, E., et al. "Understanding Economic and Other Burdens of Terminal Illness: The Experience of Patients and Their Caregivers." *Annals of Internal Medicine* 132, no. 6 (March 21, 2000): 451–459.

"Emerging Scientific Knowledge about Minimally Conscious States." *Initiatives* 22 (October 2004): 5.

Ethics and Humanities Subcommittee of the American Academy of Neurology. "Certain Aspects of Care and Management of Profoundly and Irreversibly Paralyzed Patients with Retained Consciousness and Cognition." *Neurology* 43 (1993): 222–223.

Federal Interagency Forum on Aging-Related Statistics. *Older Americans 2004: Key Indicators of Well-Being*. http://www.agingstats.gov.

Ferrell, B. A., B. R. Ferrell, and L. Rivera. "Pain in Cognitively Impaired Nursing Home Patients." *Journal of Pain Symptom Management* 10 (1995): 591–598.

Ferrell, B. R. "Cost Issues Surrounding the Treatment of Cancer Related Pain." *Journal of Pharmaceutical Care for Pain Symptom Control* 1 (1993): 9–23.

Fine, R., and T. Mayo. "Resolution of Futility by Due Process: Early Experience with the Texas Advance Directive Act." *Annals of Internal Medicine* 138 (2003): 743–746.

"Five Wishes." *Aging With Dignity* (March 6, 2007): 1–2. http://www.agingwithdignity.org/5wishes.html.

Foley, K. M. "Controlling Cancer Pain." *Hospital Practice* 121 (April 15, 2000): 101–112.

"*Foubister v. Oregon*: Doctor Cited for Negligence for Undertreating Pain." *American Medical News* (September 27, 1999): 7, 9.

Freer, J. "Brain Death." In *Ethics Committee Core Curriculum*, University of Buffalo Center for Clinical Ethics and Humanities in Health Care (December 14, 2001): 1–2. http://wings.buffalo.edu/faculty/research/bioethics/man-deth.html.

Galton, F. "Statistical Inquiries into the Efficacy of Prayer." *Fortnightly Review* 18 (1872): 125–135.

Gartner, J., D. B. Larson, and G. D. Allen. "Religious Commitment and Mental Health: A Review of the Empirical Literature." *Journal of Psychology and Theology* 19 (1991): 6–25.

Gilgunn v. Massachusetts Hospital, SUCV92-4820 (Massachusetts Superior Court, Suffolk County, April 21, 1995).

Grady, D. "Medical and Ethical Questions Raised on Deaths of Critically Ill Patients," New York Times, July 20, 2006. http://www.nytimes.com/2006/07/20/health/20ethics.html.

Grant, E. R. "Medical Futility: Legal and Ethical Aspects." *Law, Medicine and Health Care* 20 (1992): 330–335.

Griener, G. G. "The Physician's Authority to Withhold Futile Treatment." *Journal of Medicine and Philosophy* 20 (April 1995): 207–223.

Gula, R. *Reason Informed by Faith*. New York: Paulist Press, 1989.

———. "Spirituality and Ethics in Healthcare." *Health Progress* 4 (July–August 2000): 17–19.

Haig, A. J., and J. M. Ruess. "Recovery from Vegetative State of Six Months' Duration Associated with Sinemet (levodopa/carbidopa)." *Archives of Physical Medicine and Rehabilitation* 7 (1990): 1081–1083.

Halevy, A., and B. Brody. "Brain Death: Reconciling Definitions, Criteria, and Tests." *Annals of Internal Medicine* 119, no. 6 (September 15, 1993): 519–525. http://www.annals.org/cgi/content/full/119/6/519.

———. "The Houston Process-Based Approach to Medical Futility." *Bioethics Forum* 14 (Summer 1998): 10–17.

Hamel, R. and M. Panicola. "Must We Preserve Life?" *America* 190 (2004): 6–13.

Hampton, T. "Researchers Probe Pathways of Pain." *Journal of the American Medical Association* 290, no. 18 (November 12, 2003): 2391–2392.

Harold, E. "Outside the Community." *Hastings Center Report* 22 (November–December 1992): 32–35.

Hazinski, M. F., et al. "Major Changes in 2005 AHA Guidelines for CPR and ECC." *Circulation* 112 (2005): IV, 206–211. http://circ.ahajournals.org/cgi/content/full/112/24_suppl/IV-206.

Hill, C. S. "When Will Adequate Pain Treatment Be the Norm?" *Journal of the American Medical Association* 274 (1995): 1881–1882.

Hippocrates, "On the Art." In Jones, W. H. S., trans., *Hippocrates*, vol. 2. Cambridge, MA: Harvard University Press, 1981.

Hippocrates. "The Art." Reprinted in Reiser, S. J., A. J. Dyck, and W. J. Curran, eds., *Ethics in Medicine*. Cambridge, MA: MIT Press, 1977.

Hoose, B. *Proportionalism: The American Debate and Its European Roots.* Washington, DC: Georgetown University Press, 1987.

"Hospice Facts and Statistics." *Hospice Association of America* (Washington, DC: 2006): 1–11. http://www.nahc.org/Consumer/hpcstats.html.

"Hospice Fact Sheet." *National Cancer Institute* (2006): 1–4. http://www.cancer.gov/cancertopics/factsheet/Support/hospice.

"Hospice, Palliative and End of Life Care Statistics." *About.Com: Palliative Care* (November 27, 2006) 1–2. http://dying.about.com/od/hospicecare/ss/hospice_stats.htm.

Illinois Bishops. "Facing the End of Life." *Origins* 31 (June 21, 2001): 106–109.

Institute of Medicine, *Approaching Death: Improving Care at the End of Life.* Washington, DC: National Academy Press, 1997.

Jansen, L., and D. Sulmasy. "Sedation, Alimentation, Hydration, and Equivocation: Careful Conversation about Care at the End of Life." *Annals of Internal Medicine* 136 (2002): 845–849.

Jecker, N., and L. Schneiderman. "Futility and Rationing." *The American Journal of Medicine* 92 (1992): 189–196.

Jenkins, B. G., et al. "Opioid Prescribing: An Assessment Using Quality Statements." *Journal of Clinical Pharmacology Therapy* 30, no. 6 (2005): 597–602.

Jennett, B. *The Vegetative State: Medical Facts, Ethical and Legal Dilemmas.* Cambridge: Cambridge University Press, 2002.

————, and F. Plum. "Persistent Vegetative State after Brain Damage: A Syndrome in Search of a Name." *Lancet* 1 (1972): 734–737.

John Paul II. "Care for Patients in a Persistent Vegetative State." *Origins* 33 (2004): 739–752.

————. *Evangelium Vitae* no. 65, *Origins* 24 (1995): 687–727.

Joint Commission of Catholic Bishops' Conferences. "Order for the Blessing of Adults." In *Book of Blessings.* New York: Catholic Book Publishing, 1989.

Joint Commission on Accreditation of Healthcare Organizations. *Comprehensive Accreditation Manual for Hospitals: The Official Handbook* (August 1999): RI.1.2.8.

Jones, J. H. *Bad Blood: The Tuskegee Syphilis Experiment—a Tragedy of Race and Medicine.* New York: The Free Press, 1981.

————. "The Tuskegee Legacy: AIDS and the Black Community." *Hastings Center Report* 22 (November–December 1992): 38–40.

Jonsen, A., R. Veatch, and L. Walters. *Source Book in Bioethics: A Documentary History.* Washington, DC: Georgetown University Press, 1998.

Kaczor, C. "Double-Effect Reasoning from Jean Pierre Gury to Peter Knauer." *Theological Studies* 59 (1998): 297–316.

Kalina, K. "Hope for the Journey: Meaningful Support for the Terminally Ill." In *Respect Life.* Washington DC: United States Conference of Catholic Bishops, 2001.

Katchadourian, H., "Is the Principle of Double Effect Morally Acceptable?" *International Philosophical Quarterly* 27 (1988): 21–30.

Keenan, J. "The Function of the Principle of Double Effect." *Theological Studies* 54 (1993): 294–315.

Kelleher, M. M. "Ritual." In Komonchak, J., M. Collins, and D. Lane, eds., *The New Dictionary of Theology*. Collegeville, MN: Liturgical Press, 1987 (906–907).

Kelly, G. *Medico-Moral Problems*. St. Louis, MO: The Catholic Health Association of the United States and Canada, 1957.

————. "The Duty of Using Artificial Means of Preserving Life." *Theological Studies* 11 (1950): 203–220.

Kidder, D. "The Effects of Hospice Coverage on Medicare Expenditures." *Health Services Research* 117 (1992): 599–606.

King, P. A. "The Dangers of Difference." *Hastings Center Report* 22 (November–December 1992): 35–38.

Knauer, P. "*La détermination du bien et du mal moral par le principe de double effet*." *Nouvelle revue théologique* 87 (1965): 356–76.

Kübler-Ross, E. *On Death and Dying*. New York: Macmillan, 1969.

Kuczewski, M. "Talking about Spirituality in the Clinical Setting: Can Being Professional Require Being Personal?" Address given at the University of Pittsburgh (March 2007): 1–22. http://www.pitt.edu/~cep/calendar.html.

LaGanga, M., and T. Monmaney. "Doctor Found Liable in Suit over Pain." *Los Angeles Times* (June 15, 2001): A-1, A-34.

Landau, R. L., and J. M. Gustafson. "Death Is Not the Enemy." *Journal of the American Medical Association*, 252, no. 17 (1984): 2458.

Larsson, B. A. "Pain Management in Neonates." *Acta Paediatrica* 88 (1999): 1301–1310.

Lazar, N., et al. "Bioethics for Clinicians: 24. Brain Death." *Canadian Medical Association Journal* 164, no. 6 (March 20, 2001): 833–836.

Lo, B., et al. "Discussing Religious and Spiritual issues at the End of Life." *Journal of the American Medical Association* 287, no. 6 (February 13, 2002): 749–754.

Luce, J. M. "Physicians Do Not Have a Responsibility to Provide Futile or Unreasonable Care If a Patient or Family Insists." *Critical Care Medicine* 23 (1995): 761.

Lynn, J. *Sick to Death and Not Going to Take It Anymore!* Berkeley: University of California Press, 2004.

———, and D. Adamson. "Living Well at the End of Life: Adapting Health Care to Serious Chronic Illness in Old Age." Washington, DC: Rand, 2003   (1–21).   http//www.rand.org/pubs/white_papers/WP137/index.html.

———, and J. Childress. "Must Patients Always Be Given Food and Water?" in Howell, J., and W. Sale, eds., *Life Choices*. Washington, DC: Georgetown University Press, 1995 (201–213).

———, et al. "Perceptions by Family Members of the Dying Experience of Older and Seriously Ill Patients." *Annals of Internal Medicine* 126 (1997): 97–106.

Manard, B., and C. Perrone. *Hospice Care: An Introduction and Review of Evidence*. Arlington, VA: National Hospice Organization, 1994.

Mangan, J. "An Historical Analysis of the Principle of Double Effect." *Theological Studies* 10 (March 1949): 39–48.

Marks, R. M., and E. J. Sachar. "Undertreatment of Medical Inpatients with Narcotic Analgesics." *Annals of Internal Medicine* 78 (1973): 173–181.

Marrone, R. "Dying, Mourning, and Spirituality: A Psychological Perspective." *Death Studies* 23 (1999): 495–519.

Mayo Clinic Staff. "Hospice Care: An Option for People with Terminal Illness." *Mayo Clinic* (April 17, 2006): 1–4. http//www.mayoclinic.com/health/hospice-care/HQ00860.

McCaffrey, A., et al. "Prayer for Health Concerns." *Archives of Internal Medicine* 164 (April 26, 2004): 858–862.

McCormick, R. A., S.J. *Corrective Vision: Explorations in Moral Theology.* Kansas City, KS: Sheed & Ward, 1994.

———. *Health and Medicine in the Catholic Tradition.* New York: Crossroad, 1984.

———. *Notes on Moral Theology: 1965 through 1980.* Washington, DC: University Press of America, 1981.

———. "To Save or Let Die: The Dilemma of Modern Medicine." In *How Brave a New World?: Dilemmas in Bioethics.* Washington, DC: Georgetown University Press, 1981.

———, and P. Ramsey, eds. *Doing Evil to Achieve Good.* Chicago, IL: Loyola University Press, 1978.

"MCW Researchers Identify Steps to Improve CPR Survival." Medical College of Wisconsin (2004): 1–2. http://healthlink.mcw.edu/article/1031002362.html.

Medical Consultants on the Diagnosis of Death to the President's Commission for the Study of Ethical Problems in Medicine and Biomedical and Behavioral Research. "Guidelines for the Determination of Death." *Journal of the American Medical Association* 246, no. 19 (November 13, 1981): 2184–2186.

Meldrum, M. "A Capsule History of Pain Management." *Journal of the American Medical Association* 290, no. 18 (November 12, 2003): 2470–2475.

Merskey, H., and N. Bogduk, eds. *Classification of Chronic Pain*, 2nd ed. Seattle, WA: IASP Press, 1994.

Miller, M. "Making Decisions about Advance Health Care Directives." In Hamel, R., ed., *Making Health Care Decisions: A Catholic Guide.* Liguori, MO: Liguori, 2006 (91–108).

Modjarrad, K. "Medicine and Spirituality." *Journal of the American Medical Association* 291, no. 23 (January 16, 2004): 2880.

Morioka, M. "Reconsidering Brain Death: A Lesson from Japan's Fifteen Years Experience." *Hastings Center Report* 31, no. 4 (2001): 41–46.

Morrison, R. S., and D. Meier. "Palliative Care." *New England Journal of Medicine* 350, no. 25 (June 17, 2004): 2582–2590.

Multi-Society Task Force on PVS. "Medical Aspects of the Persistent Vegetative State—First of Two Parts." *New England Journal of Medicine* 330 (1994): 1499–1508.

———. "Medical Aspects of the Persistent Vegetative State—Second of Two Parts." *New England Journal of Medicine* 330 (1994): 1572–1779.

Mulvihill, N. "Giving Patients a 'Good Death.'" *Health Progress* 85, no. 4 (July–August 2004): 23–26.

National Commission for the Protection of Human Subjects of Biomedical and Behavioral Research. *The Belmont Report: Ethical Principles and Guidelines for the Protection of Human Subjects of Research.* Washington, DC: U.S. Government Printing Office, 1979.

National Hospice and Palliative Care Organization. *Hospice Care: A Physician's Guide.* Alexandria, VA: National Hospice and Palliative Care Organization, 1998.

"New Medication for Cancer Breakthrough Pain." *The National Pain Foundation* (November 21, 2006): 1–2. http://www.nationalpainfoundation.org/MyTreatment/News_Fentora.asp.

"NHPCO's Facts and Figures—2005 Findings." *National Hospice and Palliative Care Organization* (November 2006): 1–3. http://www.nhpco.org/files/public/2005-facts-and-figures.pdf.

O'Hara, D. "Is There a Role for Prayer and Spirituality in Health Care?" *Medical Clinics of North America* 86, no. 1 (January 2002): 33–46.

Okie, S. "Doctor's Duty to Ease Pain at Issue in California Lawsuit." *Washington Post* (May 7, 2001): A-3.

Olick, R. S. "Brain Death, Religious Freedom, and Public Policy." *Kennedy Institute of Ethics Journal* 1, no. 4 (1991): 275–288.

Olive, K. "Religion and Spirituality: Important Variables Frequently Ignored in Clinical Research." *Southern Medical Association* 97, no. 12 (December 2004): 1152.

O'Rourke, K., and P. Boyle. "Tissue Transplantation." In *Medical Ethics: Sources of Catholic Teachings*, 3rd ed. Washington, DC: Georgetown University Press, 1999.

Panicola, M. "Catholic Teaching on Prolonging Life: Setting the Record Straight." *Hastings Center Report* 31 (2001): 14–25.

Paris, J., and R. McCormick. "The Catholic Tradition on the Use of Nutrition and Fluids." *America* 156 (1987): 356–361.

Pellegrino, E. D. "Christ, Physician and Patient, the Model for Christian Healing." *The Linacre Quarterly* 66 (August 1999): 70–78.

————, and D. C. Thomasma. *A Philosophical Basis of Medical Practice.* New York: Oxford University Press, 1981.

Pennsylvania Department of Health. "Out-of-Hospital Do-Not-Resuscitate (DNR) Orders: A Guide for Patients and Families" (January 26, 2007): 1–2. http://www.dsf.health.state.pa.us/health/cwp/view.asp?a=170& Q=234321.

Pennsylvania Legislature. "Act 169 of 2006—Pennsylvania Health Care Decision Making," Title 20, Chapter 54, Pa. C.S.A. Sections 5421– 5488. http://www2.legis.state.pa.us/WU01/LI/BI/BT/2005/0/SB0628 P2117.pdf.

Pennsylvania Medical Society. "Advance Health Care Directives and Health Care Decision-Making for Incompetent Patients: A Guide to Act 169 of 2006 for Physicians and Other Health Care Providers" (2006). http://www.pamedsoc.org.

Pius XII. "The Prolongation of Life." *The Pope Speaks* 4 (1958): 395–396.

Place, M. "Thoughts on the Papal Allocution." *Health Progress* 85 (2004): 6, 60.

Poloma, M. M., and B. F. Pendleton. "The Effects of Prayer and Prayer Experiences on Measures of General Well-Being." *Journal of Psychology and Theology* 19 (1991): 71–93.

Porter, J., and H. Jick. "Addiction Rare in Patients Treated with Narcotics." *New England Journal of Medicine* 320 (1980): 123.

Powner, D. J., B. M. Ackerman, and A. Grenvik. "Medical Diagnosis of Death in Adults: Historical Contributions to Current Controversies." *Lancet* 348 (1996): 1219–1223.

President's Commission for the Study of Ethical Problems in Medicine and Biomedical and Behavioral Research. "Defining Death: A Report on the Medical, Legal and Ethical Issues in the Determination of Death." Washington, DC: U.S. Government Printing Office, 1981.

President's Council on Bioethics. *Taking Care: Ethical Caregiving in Our Aging Society* (September 2005). http://www.bioethics.gov.

Quality Standards Subcommittee of the American Academy of Neurology. "Practice Parameters: Assessment and Management of Patients in a Persistent Vegetative State." *Neurology* 45 (1995): 1015–1018.

Relecciones Theologicas, edition critica. Madrid: Imprenta La Rafa, vol. 3, 1933–1935.

Rich, B. A. "An Ethical Analysis of the Barriers to Effective Pain Management." *Cambridge Quarterly of Healthcare Ethics* 9 (2000): 54–70.

———. "Pain Management: Legal Risks and Ethical Responsibilities." *Journal of Pharmaceutical Care in Pain Symptom Control* 5 (1997): 5–20.

Ringold, S., and T. Glass. "Cardiopulmonary Resuscitation (CPR)." *Journal of the American Medical Association* 293 (January 19, 2005): 388.

Rubenstein, A., E. Cohen, and E. Jackson. "The Definition of Death and the Ethics of Organ Procurement from the Deceased," Discussion paper for the President's Council on Bioethics (September 2006): 1–35. http://bioethicsprint.bioethics.gov/background/runenstein.html.

Sacred Congregation for the Doctrine of the Faith. "Declaration on Euthanasia" part IV. *Origins* 10 (1980): 154–157.

Satel, A. "Doctors Behind Bars: Treating Pain Is Now Risky Business." *New York Times* (October 19, 2004): 1–3. http://www.nytimes.com/2004/10/19/health/policy/19essa.html.

Schneiderman, L., N. Jecker, and A. Jonsen. "Medical Futility: Its Meaning and Ethical Implications." *Annals of Internal Medicine* 112 (June 15, 1990): 949–950.

―――. "Medical Futility: Response to Critiques." *Annals of Internal Medicine* 125 (October 15, 1996): 669–674.

Schnitzer, T. J. "Non-NSAID Pharmacologic Treatment Options for the Management of Chronic Pain." *American Journal of Medicine* 105 (1998): 45S–52S.

Schüller, B. "The Double Effect in Catholic Thought: A Reevaluation." In McCormick, R., and P. Ramsey, eds., *Doing Evil to Achieve Good*. Chicago, IL: Loyola University Press, 1978 (165–191).

Sengstaken, E. A., and S. A. King, "The Problems of Pain and Its Detection among Geriatric Nursing Home Residents." *Journal of the American Geriatric Society* 41 (1993): 541–544.

Shannon, T., and J. Walter. "Artificial Nutrition, Hydration: Assessing Papal Statement." *National Catholic Reporter* 4 (2004): 1–4.

Shaw, J. "POLST: Honoring Wishes at the End of Life." *Health Care Ethics USA* 15, no. 1 (Winter 2007): 1–17.

Sheehan, M. "Feeding Tubes: Sorting Out the Issues." *Health Progress* 6 (2001): 22–27.

————. "A Great Comfort." *America* (October 7, 2000): 8–11.

————. "On Dying Well." *America* (July 29–August 5, 2000): 12–15.

Slack, J., and M. Faut-Callahan. "Pain Management." *Clinical Nursing in North America* 26 (1991): 463–476.

Sloan, R. P., E. Bagiella, and T. Powell. "Religion, Spirituality, and Medicine." *Lancet* 353 (1999): 664–667.

"The Slow Code—Should Anyone Rush to Its Defense?" *New England Journal of Medicine* 338, no. 7 (February 12, 1998): 467–469.

Soto, D. *De Justitia et Jure* (Venice, Italy: 1568).

Sparks, R. *To Treat or Not to Treat*. New York: Paulist Press, 1988.

Steinhauser, K., et al. "In Search of a Good Death: Observations of Patients, Families, and Providers." *Annals of Internal Medicine* 132, no. 10 (May 16, 2000): 825–832.

Sternbach, R. A. "Clinical Aspects of Pain." In Sternbach, R. A., ed., *The Psychology of Pain*. New York: Raven, 1978.

Stewart, W. F., et al. "Lost Productive Time and Cost Due to Common Pain Conditions in the U.S. Workforce." *Journal of the American Medical Association* 290 (2003): 2443–2454.

Sulmasy, D. "Are Feeding Tubes Morally Obligatory?" *St. Anthony Messenger* (January 2006): 1–7. http://www.americancatholic.org/Messenger/Jan2006/Feature1.asp.

————. *The Healer's Calling: A Spirituality for Physicians and Other Health Care Professionals*. New York: Paulist Press, 1997.

SUPPORT Principle Investigators. "A Controlled Trial to Improve Care for Seriously Ill Hospitalized Patients: A Study to Understand Prognoses and Preferences for Outcomes and Risks of Treatments (SUPPORT)." *Journal of the American Medical Association* 274, no. 4 (November 22–29, 1995): 1591–1598.

Task Force for Quality at the End of Life. "Improving End-of-Life Experiences for Pennsylvanians" (February 5, 2007): 1–39.http://www.aging.state.pa.us.

Task Force on Pain Management—Catholic Health Association. "Pain Management: Theological and Ethical Principles Governing the Use of Pain Relief for Dying Patients." *Health Progress* (January–February 1993): 30–39, 65.

Taylor, P. "Hospice: Caring When There Is No Cure." *Advance for Nurses* (February 1, 1999): 20.

Teno, J. M., et al. "Family Perspectives on End-of-Life Care at the Last Place of Care." *Journal of the American Medical Association* 291, no. 1 (January 7, 2004): 88–93.

———. "Research Letter: Persistent Pain in Nursing Home Residents." *Journal of the American Medical Association* 285, no. 16 (April 25, 2001): 2081.

Texas Catholic Bishops and the Texas Conference of Catholic Health Care Facilities. "On Withdrawing Artificial Nutrition and Hydration." *Origins* 20 (1990): 53–55.

Tolle, S. W., et al. "A Prospective Study of the Efficacy of the Physician Order Form for Life-Sustaining Treatment." *Journal of the American Geriatrics Society* 46, no. 9 (September 1998): 1097–1102.

"Top Court OKs Assisted-Suicide Law." *MSNBC* (January 18, 2006):1–2. http://www.msnbc.msn.com/id/10891536/print/q/displaymode/1098.

Trafford, A. "No Pain Relief for Some: Study Points Out Inequality in Care." *Philadelphia Inquirer* (September 4, 2000), E-3.

Trau, J., and J. McCartney. "In the Best Interest of the Patient." *Health Progress* (April 1993): 50–56.

Uniform Definition of Death Act. 12 Uniform Laws Annotated 320 (1990 Supp). See also "Uniform Definition of Death Act," *Journal of the*

American Medical Association 246, no. 19 (November 13, 1981): 2184–2186.

United States Catholic Conference of Bishops. *Ethical and Religious Directives for Catholic Health Care Services*, 4th ed. Washington, DC: U.S. Catholic Conference of Bishops, 2001.

United States Catholic Conference of Bishops. *Ethical and Religious Directives for Catholic Health Care Services*, 5th ed. Washington, DC: U.S. Catholic Conference of Bishops, 2009

United States Congress. "Federal Patient Self-Determination Act of 1990." 42 U.S.C. 1395 cc (a) subpart E, section 4751. http://www.fha.org/acrobat/patientselfdetermination_act_1990.pdf.

Vacco v. Quill, 65 *U.S. Law Wk.* 4695, 117 S. Ct. 2293 (1997).

Vastag, B. "Scientists Find Connections in the Brain between Physical and Emotional Pain." *Journal of the American Medical Association* 290, no. 18 (November 12, 2003): 2389–2390.

Vitz, M. "Let Us Not Forsake the Dying, Says Pa. Report." *Philadelphia Inquirer* (February 5, 2007): 1–2. http://www.philly.com/mld/inquirer/16623894.htm?template=contentModules/printstory.jsp.

Waldman, H. "A Last Compassion Resisted." *Hartford Courant* (January 29, 2006): 1, 44.

Walter, J. J. "Proportionate Reason and Its Three Levels of Inquiry: Structuring the Ongoing Debate." *Louvain Studies* 10 (Spring 1984): 32.
———, and T. Shannon. "Implications of the Papal Allocution on Tube Feeding." *Hastings Center Report* 34 (2004): 18–20.

Washington v. Glucksberg, 65 *U.S. Law Wk.* 4669, 117 S. Ct. 2258 (1997).

Weiner, R. S. "An Interview with John J. Bonica, M.D." *Pain Practitioner* 1 (1989): 2.

Wertheimer, P., M. Jouvet, and J. Descotes. "A Propos du Diagnostic de la Mort du Système Nerveux les Comas avec Arrêt Respiratoire Traités par Respiration Artificielle." *Presse Med* 67 (1959): 87–88.

"What is Hospice?" *American Cancer Society* (August 2004): 1–4. http://www.cancer.org/docroot/eto/content/eto_2_5x_what_is_hospice_care.asp?

Wik, L., et al. "Quality of Cardiopulmonary Resuscitation during Out-of-Hospital Cardiac Arrest." *Journal of the American Medical Association* 293 (January 19, 2005): 299–304.

Wildes, K. "Ordinary and Extraordinary Means and the Quality of Life." Theological Studies 57 (1996): 500–512.

Wirth, D. P., and B. J. Mitchell. "Complementary Healing Therapy for Patients with Type-1 Diabetes Milletus." Journal of Scientific Exploration 8 (1994): 367–377.

Working Group of the Royal College of Physicians. "The Permanent Vegetative State." Journal of the Royal College of Physicians 30 (1996): 119–121.

World Health Organization. "Definition of Palliative Care" (1990). http://www.who.int/cancer/paliative/definition/en/. Retrieved on December 12, 2006.

Younger, S. J., et al. "'Brain Death' and Organ Retrieval: A Cross Sectional Survey and Concepts among Health Professionals." Journal of the American Medical Association 261 (1989): 2205–2210.

INDEX

A

abandonment, fear of, 186–188
acceptance of death, 186, 188–190
Ackerman, Felicia, 156
acute pain, 117–118, 121
Acute Physiology and Chronic Health Evaluation (APACHE) system, 211 n 28
addiction, fear of, 118, 125–127
Adult Medical Futility Policy, 55–59
Adult Palliative Care: Policy and Procedure, 67–70
advance directives/living wills, 77–85, 201
Aetna, 154
affirmation of individuality, 4
allocutions, purpose of, 34–35
allow natural death (AND) order, 75, 97
American Academy of Neurology, 14, 15, 32
American Academy of Pediatrics, 14
American Association of Neurological Surgeons, 14
American Medical Association, 33, 118
AND (allow natural death) order, 75, 97
anesthesia, 24, 117
APACHE (Acute Physiology and Chronic Health Evaluation) system, 211 n 28
Aquinas, Thomas, 23, 131
artificial nutrition and hydration
    as burden, 23, 29
    considered obligatory, 28
    and fear of suffering, 17, 18
    and John Paul II's allocation, 29–34
    as "normal care," 30
    See also ordinary-extraordinary means distinction
Aspen Criteria, 15
aspirin, 118
attending physician, defined, 79
autonomy, Christian view of, 48

autonomy of patients, 46–47, 50–51, 128–129
awareness, 13, 14, 15–16

B

Baby K case (1994), 40
"bad deaths," characteristics of, 2–3
bad news, steps for delivering, 6–7
Bañez, Domingo, 23, 24
Basil the Great, 22
Bayberry Care Center, Tomlinson v., 215 n 23
Bayer Company, 118
beneficence, 48, 50–51, 129
Benson, Herbert, 180–181
Bergman, William, 215 n 23
brain death diagnosis, 10–13, 18–19
brain disorders, 10–13, 206 n 28
brain injury, 206 n 28
brain lesions, 15–16
breakthrough pain, 126–127
breathing difficulties, 163–164
Brody, Baruch, 46
Brother Fox case (1979), 71
burdens, excessive, 23–24, 25–26, 33
Byrd, R.C., 180

C

Campbell, J.D., 181, 183
cardiopulmonary resuscitation (CPR), 73–74
"Care for Patients in a Permanent Vegetative State" (John Paul II), 21, 30
care given in terminal situation, 3
Catholic health care facilities, ethical issues faced by, 36–37, 51–52
Catholic teaching on ordinary-extraordinary means distinction, 20–21
Cephalon, 127

245